MEDICAL MARIJUANA
DESK REFERENCE

FIRST EDITION

ALICIA K. WILBUR, PHD

LORI J. GLAUSER, MBA

FOREWORD BY

DAVID M. SIPPER, MD

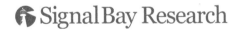

Subsidiary of Signal Bay, Inc. (OTC: SGBY)

Medical Marijuana Desk Reference, First Edition
Published by

Signal Bay Research
Division of Signal Bay, Inc. (OTC: SGBY)
9484 S. Eastern Ave #141
Las Vegas, NV 89123
www.signalbayinc.com

Disclaimer

Marijuana is illegal under US federal law, and the laws of most nations worldwide.

Under US federal law, the controlled substances act regulates, among other things, the possession and distribution of certain controlled substances including cannabis. This also applies in states that have enacted cannabis laws for medical purposes or for adult use. This book describes the medical research that has been performed to date, and has been performed under tightly controlled conditions and with stringent regulation.

Some US states and some nations permit the use of medical marijuana under highly regulated conditions and with the referral of a qualified physician. Summaries of federal and state marijuana laws and regulations are available at www.cannaiq.com. Please refer to seek professional legal advice with regards to consuming, providing, or recommending cannabis. For a listing of qualifying medical conditions by state, refer to www.mmdr.co.

The Medical Marijuana Desk Reference does not provide medical advice

The contents of the Medical Marijuana Desk Reference ("MMDR") is for informational purposes only. While we strive to provide you factual data reflecting peer reviewed research studies, the content is not intended to be a substitute for professional medical advice, diagnosis, or treatment. Always seek the advice of your physician or other qualified health providers with any questions you may have regarding a medical condition. Never, under any conditions, disregard professional medical advice or delay in seeking it because of something you have read in this manual.

If you think you may have a medical emergency, call your physician or dial 911 immediately. The publisher and authors of this book do not recommend or endorse any specific products, procedures, opinions, or other information that may be mentioned in the book. Reliance on any information provided by the Medical Marijuana Desk Reference, cannaIQ.com, Signal Bay Inc., or its employees or affiliates is solely at your own risk, and we are not responsible for any actions taken with the information we provide.

For general information on our other products and services, please contact Signal Bay Inc. at (888) 978-5066 or email customercare@signalbayinc.com.

CONTENTS

List of Tables

About the Author

ALICIA K. WILBUR, PHD. has been a scientist, teacher, and writer since 1997. Her specialization and main areas of interest are evolution and human disease. She holds undergraduate degrees in anthropology and biology from Indiana University and a Ph.D. in biological anthropology from The University of New Mexico. She has been the recipient of a National Science Foundation Graduate Research Fellowship, a National Science Foundation Doctoral Dissertation Improvement grant, and a Wenner-Gren Foundation grant. She was a Postdoctoral Research Scientist at Arizona State University, and a Research Scientist at the University of Washington. Dr. Wilbur has taught courses on human evolution, human skeletal anatomy, human biological variation, and the co-evolution of humans and infectious diseases at The University of New Mexico, Arizona State University, and University of Washington. She is an author of several peer-reviewed articles in scientific journals, as well as a college textbook on disease and human evolution. She has lectured on subjects including the evolution of tuberculosis and leprosy throughout the United States, and in Canada, England, Paraguay, and Taiwan. Dr. Wilbur's current interests include the utility of medicinal marijuana in the treatment of debilitating conditions.

LORI J. GLAUSER, MBA is co-founder and President of Signal Bay Research and provided the inspiration for this book. Ms. Glauser has over 20 years' experience in management consulting, industry research, engineering, and startups, and has expertise in business planning, business process design, financial forecasting, risk, customer experience, supply chain management, and energy management. She is also creator of cannaIQ. com, a website that provides information about the cannabis industry for professionals. She has experience with regulatory and policy issues, and has supported development of witness testimony documents. Lori has a BS in Mechanical Engineering from the University of New Hampshire and an MBA from University of Alabama. Lori was also adjunct instructor of Project Management at the Metropolitan State College of Denver.

Contributors

DAVID M. SIPPER, MD has practiced obstetrical anesthesiology and pain management for 25 years, and has been a resident of Las Vegas for 22 years. Previously, he was an Assistant Clinical Professor at UC Irvine, where he was in charge of setting up and managing the acute and chronic pain management services, and the related teaching components of the residency program. He has extensive experience working with and formulating controlled-substances, and caring for patients with chronic pain, in multi-modal settings.

Additionally, Dr. Snipper has extensive practical business experience, having set-up 8 various real estate development, contracting, consulting, management partnerships, during the time he has been in Las Vegas, as well as participating in the purchase and operations of a outpatient medical facility, a cabinet/closet business, and a swimming pool contracting business. He is always looking to create new concepts in business/medicine that will be of benefit to patients and communities. He has also served on the Board of a synagogue and a charitable art foundation. Currently, he is a principal of several licensed medical marijuana establishments in Las Vegas, and is bringing together industry, patient, and healthcare-realated groups, in order to better serve the industry.

EDWARD J. ABRAVANEL is a cannabis cultivation expert and cannabis industry pioneer. He founded the first medical marijuana dispensary in Detroit, and produced a line of edible products called "Ed's Meds". Mr. Abravanel is a graduate of Oaksterdam University.

Acknowledgments

We would like to acknowledge all those who contributed to the production of this book. Jeannee Vale, massage therapist and healthcare advocate, worked tirelessly to assist in editing and making the work accessible to even nonscientists. Eddie Abravanel, a master grower and cannabis aficionado and Kristin Neuenschwander from Advanced CRA Consulting provided valuable insight into the world of the cannabis. Laura Seo, Harvard University student assisted with our research.

We would like to acknowledge the hundreds of scientists and physicians who studied this plant, many of whom did so when placed against tremendous legal and logistical hurdles to perform the research.

Most of all we would like to acknowledge the thousands of brave patients and their families who in some cases take great risk to participate in these studies for the betterment of the understanding of medical cannabis.

Finally, we would like to dedicate this work to all the patients, their families, and other caregivers who have benefitted from the use of this plant and who work to advocate its use for other patients.

FOREWORD

With recent widespread political push from the people across the United States to legalize the use of cannabis, for medicinal and recreational use, many states, in advance of the federal government, have passed laws. The ensuing chaos has made for interesting reading, but also for some unique opportunities. It is rare that individuals from the science and healthcare fields can participate in the early growth of an industry, at least in part due to the perception that the risks taken in such participation are something not ordinarily a part of "professional conduct." Opportunities in the cannabis industry are exciting because we are dealing with a plant that was first viewed as medicine; in fact has been viewed as such throughout written history. Its reappearance, then, demands careful scientific examination, as to its medicinal uses and effectiveness, its safety, and its potential future contribution to healthcare and health management in general.

The first logical step for scientists is to perform a careful search of the currently existing literature; next to compile and audit this compilation; and then to summarize and present the results of such review process in the form of a compendium that is clear, concise, well-organized, and easy to read and understand. Dr. Alicia Wilbur has done just that in creating this Medical Marijuana Desk Reference. While Dr. Wilbur refers to this text as merely an "introduction," the book in fact delves rather deeply into the important aspects of the history of the cannabis plant, and then presents an excellent review of the botany of the plant and the physiology and pharmacology of the cannabinoids, and then transitions through a summary of delivery systems and physiological effects. I must tell the reader that as a physician, I am amazed that I had to learn much of this basic information through texts such as this, as opposed to part of a medical school curriculum. Thankfully, that is starting to change.

The heart of the book consists of a complete description of cannabis uses and effects, along with related literature as may be available, classified by diseases and disease states, and also by reviews of which states currently allow which particular uses. And where there are documented negative effects, these are presented as well. And references are provided.

It is incredible to note that there are over 80 diseases and/or symptom complexes for which cannabis has been shown by scientific evidence to be of definitive human benefit. And I imagine that more will be determined as the many research projects around the nation bear fruit.

For a patient or a caregiver with a family member facing chronic or critical illness, the cannabis novice, aficionado, physician, scientist, or otherwise, Dr. Wilbur's Desk Reference is a "user-friendly" manual that I hope will find its way into the homes and offices of many folks who wish to have a more scientific view of the nature and value of this extraordinary plant. And I imagine that Dr. Wilbur will continue to educate us through future publications.

David M. Sipper, MD

CHAPTER 1

INTRODUCTION

C annabis (also known as marijuana) is a genus of flowering plants that originates from Central and South Asia and was domesticated at least 7000 years ago for its fibers, oil, and protein-rich seeds,[1] as well as for its medicinal and psychoactive properties.[2] In modern times, cannabis is one of the most widely distributed cultivated plants.[2] There is physical evidence of hemp fiber usage in China that may even date back 12,000 years,[3] and cannabis was reputedly used medicinally for some 5000 years.[4,5] In ancient Egypt, cannabis was used to treat conditions such as inflammation of the eye, infected toes or fingers, diarrhea, pain, and even tumors, with written evidence potentially dating as early as 2350 BC[3] Although it is uncertain, there seems to be evidence (summarized by Russo,[3]) for the ancient Mesopotamian use of cannabis to treat impotence, neuralgia, lung congestion, depression, anxiety, epilepsy, spasticity, and inflammation of the skin, and in ancient India, to treat depression. Pollen samples confirm that cannabis was present in sub-Saharan Africa at least 2000 years ago.

At least two archaeological excavations provide evidence for the use of cannabis for its psychoactive and/or medicinal properties in human cultures from as early as 3200 years ago. In the Xinjiang Uygur Autonomous Region of Northwest China, an area with a documented human presence of potentially up to 40,000 years, the tomb of a middle-aged male who is thought to have been a shaman contained a basket of vegetal remains of what appeared to be cannabis.[1] Botanical, phytochemical, and DNA analysis confirmed that this approximately 11 grams of material was indeed *Cannabis sativa* that had been processed and probably cultivated (rather than gathered from wild plants) for their high THC content. Interestingly, the authors report that no male cannabis plant parts were found – male cannabis components do not have the same degree of psychoactive properties as female parts. The fact that the tombs did not contain any hemp artifacts (such as rope or textile) supports the researchers' hypothesis that cannabis was used for its psychoactive properties in this context.

An archaeological excavation of skeletal remains near modern Jerusalem dated to AD 315-392 found evidence for cannabis use,[6] potentially to aid in the birth process. The skeleton was of an adolescent female, and the pelvic region contained a skeletal fetus that would have been too large to be birthed vaginally – in the same abdominal area of the skeleton was found a grey, carbonized material that was microscopically identified as cannabis. Further analysis by thin-layer chromatography identified the cannabis compound THC, which is thought to have been burned to facilitate (unfortunately, unsuccessfully in this case) birth. By the ninth century A.D. cannabis was used by Islamic physicians to treat helminthic worm infestations and neuropathic pain.[3] According to Russo,[3] publication of the experimentally verified benefits of cannabis to cure the plague brought about widespread medical usage of cannabis in Europe and North America by the mid-nineteenth century. At that time, parts of the cannabis plant became a common treatment for conditions such as corns, asthma, skin inflammation, incontinence, and sexually transmitted diseases.[7]

Mikuriya[8] reviews the use of cannabis as a substitute for alcohol, opiates, and other substances that were perceived as relatively more harmful during the nineteenth and early twentieth centuries. He quotes two different government reports that recommended against suppressing the use of cannabis for fear its unavailability would cause people to turn to other, more deleterious, drugs. He discusses several reports that indicate that cannabis was an effective treatment for delirium tremens (a severe mental and nervous system withdrawal symptom following cessation of alcohol during advanced alcoholism) and for withdrawal symptoms from opiates. Following prohibition of cannabis in the United States, a synthetic cannabinoid, "pyrahexyl",[9] was reported to ease alcohol withdrawal symptoms.[8]

Until 1937, cannabis was legally prescribed by US physicians for medical conditions. According to the US National Cancer Institute at the National Institutes of Health (www.cancer.gov), the Marijuana Tax Act of 1937 imposed a $1 per ounce tax for use of medical cannabis and a $100 per ounce tax for recreational use. The American Medical Association (AMA) opposed the tax for several reasons, including that physicians would have to pay a special tax just for prescribing cannabis. Additionally, Dr. William C. Woodward testified before the US House of Representatives (transcript of testimony available online at http://www.druglibrary.org/schaffer/hemp/taxact/woodward.htm) that the AMA did not believe there was objective evidence that cannabis was harmful, and that passing the act would limit research into its use as a medicine. Unfortunately, the Marihuana Tax Act was not only passed in 1937, but continued concerns about cannabis's potential for harm subsequently led to the passage of various federal laws that successively restricted possession and distribution of marijuana. These culminated in the Controlled Substance Act of 1970 (Pub. L. No. 91-513, 84 Stat. 1236 [Oct. 27, 1970]). This act ultimately classified cannabis as a Schedule I drug, a classification that is defined by high potential for abuse and no accepted medical use due to a lack of accepted safety for its use.[7] Because of the federal prohibition of cannabis use, scientific testing has been limited. In turn, limitation on scientific studies allowed the Drug Enforcement Administration to reject proposals for reassignment of cannabis as a Schedule II drug due to lack of scientific evidence for its medical efficacy. Additionally, the national "zero-tolerance" policy toward illegal drugs framed cannabis as a "gateway drug" that leads to the abuse of more deleterious drugs. Legalization of cannabis for medical purposes was thought to be a slippery slope that would lead to increased recreational use of the drug and a perception of it as "harmless," particularly among children.[7]

Despite the federal ban on cannabis, several states legalized its medical use, the first of which was California in 1996. Following years of research into the therapeutic effects of cannabis and its constituent chemicals, as well as the body's own endocannabinoid system (see Chapter 2), the Ending Federal Marijuana Prohibition Act of 2013 (H.R. 499, [Feb. 5, 2013]) was introduced to decriminalize cannabis at the federal level, granting the states the power for its regulation. In December 2014 congress passed a federal spending measure (the Consolidated and Further Continuing Appropriations Act, 2015, Section 538) which prohibits the Department of Justice from preventing states from implementing their own laws about medical marijuana use, distribution, possession, or cultivation. This measure essentially allows each state to decide the medical cannabis issue for itself. As of early 2015, 23 states and the District of Columbia have passed legislation that allows patients with certain debilitating conditions, under the care of a registered physician, to use cannabis as a treatment. An up-to-date list of condi- tions authorized by state can be found at www.medicalmarijuanadeskreference.com; website information for each state's medical cannabis program is provided in Chapter 3, Table 3.

The National Institute on Drug Abuse (NIDA, www.drugabuse.gov) indi-cates that, as of January 31, 2014, there were 28 active grants funded by NIDA to explore the potential for therapeutic use of cannabis in 6 differ-ent disease categories: autoimmune disease, inflammation, pain, psychi-atric disorder, seizures, and substance use disorders/withdrawal/depen-dence. The Medical Marijuana Desk Reference compiles primary scien-tific studies on the efficacy of marijuana for both state-authorized, and other, as yet unauthorized, conditions in an easy-to-use format. Chapter 2 describes cannabis, its active chemical constituents, the cannabinoids, and routes of administration of those. The known effects of cannabinoids on the body, especially upon the endocannabinoid system, are summa-rized, and Table 2 presents the known beneficial effects of cannabis with supporting scientific references. Chapter 3 presents authorized condi-tions by state, followed by a table of scientific references by condition according to their beneficial, detrimental, or neutral effects upon that condition. There follows a description of each medical condition and the state of scientific knowledge about the utility for that condition. Note that this report focuses solely upon natural cannabis and cannabinoids – it does not summarize the literature on synthetic cannabis or canna-binoids. Chapter 4 presents a table and discussions of other conditions for which there is scientific evidence that marijuana may be therapeutic, and the references for the evidence (again categorized into beneficial, detrimental, or neutral effects). While every effort has been made to keep the language highly readable and understandable, any report that delves into biological, medical, and general scientific literature will contain spe-cial terms. These terms have been defined throughout the text, but a glossary is also provided for easy reference. An extensive bibliography closes the report.

A scientific approach to medicine

The Medical Marijuana Desk Reference compiles information from primary scientific research published in peer-reviewed scholarly journals. "Primary scientific research" means that these are original studies performed on cannabis or cannabinoids and their effects on biological conditions, and are not anecdotal pieces, opinion pieces, or reviews (except for systematic reviews or meta-analyses, which employ sophisticated statistical techniques to analyze published studies). The vast majority of these articles were obtained by performing a search of PubMed (www.ncbi.nlm.nih.gov) using the keyword "marijuana." Opinion pieces and reviews are referenced in some cases in the text, but they are not included in the tables as works supporting the scientific efficacy of cannabis.

A scientific approach to medicine emphasizes rigorous testing of hypotheses using empirical evidence. Research may be performed using a variety of methods, including controlled experiments on human subjects or other animals, *in vitro* (outside the body, in culture or solution) studies, epidemiological studies, and systematic reviews/meta-analyses. In science, it is important that research results can be independently reproduced—results that cannot be replicated must be re-examined carefully. Scientific research is of particular importance in medicine, as health and even lives are at stake if incorrect conclusions are incorporated into practice. Scientific research builds upon the work of other researchers, and information is disseminated in a formal manner via peer-reviewed publication in an appropriate journal.

When authors send a publication to a scientific peer-reviewed journal, the paper is sent out to other experts in the field who will then carefully read and assess several aspects of the manuscript: the scientific question or hypothesis being addressed, the methods used to research the question or test the hypothesis, the results obtained, and the conclusion(s) drawn by the authors. Reviewers then recommend whether the manuscript is suitable for publication, and if so, any errors or concerns that need to be addressed. Copies of the critical reviews then go (usually anonymously) to the authors who may address the criticisms and, if the journal has accepted the manuscript for publication, return the revised manuscript for publication. The peer-review process in science is important in assessing the quality of the research and of the publication. It allows the reader, who may not be an expert in the subject of the publication, a level of assurance that the study was properly conducted, that the research methods are appropriate to the question, and that the conclusions drawn are reasonable given the results of the study and the current state of knowledge in the field. The Medical Marijuana Desk Reference is compiled from peer-reviewed scientific studies.

How to use this guide

This report is intended to introduce patients, practitioners, caregivers, dispensaries, and growers to the published scientific literature concerning the utility of cannabis as medicine. Chapter 2 gives an overview of the cannabis plant and of its biologically active components, the phytocannabinoids, or cannabinoids. It also discusses the various ways in which cannabis or cannabinoids may be administered. Table 1 presents the major individual cannabinoids that have been studied for their medicinal effects, their common abbreviations, known biological effect, and some references that summarize these effects. The numbers in the reference column correspond to the scientific references for studies of these cannabinoids. You can find the exact citation for the reference by going to the corresponding number in the bibliography at the end of the book. Bibliographic references are listed by the authors' names, year of publication, title of publication, journal in which it was published, and volume and page numbers for the article. Here is an example:

582.   Manrique-Garcia E, Zammit S, Dalman C, Hemmingsson T, Allebeck P (2012) Cannabis use and depression: a longitudinal study of a national cohort of Swedish conscripts. *BMC Psychiatry* 12:112.

582 = Reference number found in one of the tables or cited in the text

Manrique-Garcia E, Zammit S, Dalman C, Hemmingsson T, Allebeck P = **Authors' names**

(2012) = **Year of publication**

Cannabis use and depression: a longitudinal study of a national cohort of Swedish conscripts = **Title of the publication**

BMC Psychiatry = **Title of the journal**
12:112 = **Volume 12: Page 112.**

There follows a brief summary of the endocannabinoid system of the human body. This system consists of receptors in various organ systems upon which the cannabinoids made by the human body, endocannabinoids, act in various ways to regulate neurological, immune, and other functions. It is upon this endocannabinoid system that phytocannabinoids, or exocannabinoids, act to bring about medicinal effects. The known effects of cannabis on the body are summarized in Table 2, which lists the effects according to beneficial or detrimental categories, and then the associated bibliographic references. The numbers under the reference column correspond to the references in the bibliography, just as in Table 1.

Readers interested in a particular debilitating condition are referred to Chapter 3 (state-authorized conditions) and Chapter 4 (non-authorized conditions). Table 4 lists each authorized condition alphabetically and Table 5 lists each non-authorized condition alphabetically; these tables each have three columns: beneficial, neutral, and detrimental, which correspond to the conclusions the study reached about the effects of cannabis for that condition. The numbers under each column correspond to the scientific references for studies on those conditions. You can find the exact citation for the reference by going to the corresponding number in the bibliography just as in Table 1.

Following the tables of references are alphabetically organized descriptions of each condition and a brief summary of the scientific references cited in the tables. The same citation number is used in both the bibliography and in each of the tables. If you are interested in reading any of these references, look up the number in the bibliography, find the citation, and obtain it from the publisher's website or from your local library. Note that some articles may be obtained free of charge from the National Institute of Health's PubMed website (www.ncbi.nlm.nih.gov), while others require a subscription to the journal or purchase of individual articles. You may be able to find the abstract (a brief summary) of most articles on the PubMed website by searching the article or author's name.

CHAPTER 2

WHAT IS CANNABIS?

C annabis is an erect flowering herb that, in the wild, grows annually from seed. In modern times, cultivators also commonly grow the plant from clones. Cannabis is dioecious (separate plants with male and female reproductive organs), although there are also monoecious (male and female reproductive organs in a single plant) plants. There has been some controversy over the number of species in the genus Cannabis, with some suggesting that there are two or three separate species: *Cannabis sativa*, *Cannabis indica*, and *Cannabis ruderalis*, while others describe a single species, *Cannabis sativa* with variants. Cannabis contains about 70 chemicals termed "cannabinoids", at least some of which are of use pharmacologically.[10] Chemical analyses of the cannabinoids have allowed for division of Cannabis sativa varieties into the five most commonly occurring chemotypes, based upon the main cannabinoid produced at maturity and the quantity of the cannabinoids.[11]

Another generalized typing considers plants with high content of the cannabinoid THC, and low content of the cannabinoid CBD, to be marijuana, while those with low THC and high CBD are considered hemp.[2] A genome sequencing project compared the genetic profiles of the *Cannabis sativa* Purple Kush strain, used for its psychoactive and medicinal properties, with two hemp strains, Finola and USO-31, and found evidence that sufficient genetic variation exists to support a separation of marijuana species and hemp species.[2] Moreover, and perhaps unsurprisingly, the marijuana strain Purple Kush has genetic variation that causes the cells to produce more of the cannabinoids than do the hemp species. For the purposes of The Medical Marijuana Desk Reference, we will simply refer to "cannabis" and not concern ourselves with the question of species versus variety.

Phytocannabinoids are the molecules that come from plants and that can act on the cannabinoid receptors of the human body (discussed further in Chapter 3). These compounds accumulate in the female flowers (the buds) of cannabis and are known as cannabinoids.[3] As research into cannabis continues, an ever-increasing number of cannabinoids are reported in the literature.[12] Table 1 lists the main cannabinoids that have, to date, been studied for their beneficial medicinal properties. Cannabinol (CBN) was first isolated in 1895 and cannabidiol (CBD) was isolated in 1934.[13] Cannabidiol is the major non-psychoactive cannabinoid in the plant.[14] The major psychoactive compound of cannabis, delta9-tetrahydrocannabinol (THC), was first isolated in 1964.[15] Correspondingly, most of the studies that have examined the effects of individual cannabinoids (rather than the whole plant) on the body have concentrated upon these two. More information about individual cannabinoids and their effects on specific medical conditions are found in Chapters 3 and 4.

TABLE 1. Beneficial biological effects of some cannabinoids

Cannabinoid	Abbreviation	Biological effects	Scientific Reference*
Cannabichromene	CBC	Analgesic Anti-depressant Anti-diarrheal Anti-inflammation Anti-microbial Anti-proliferative	16–20
Cannabidiol	CBD	Addiction reduction Analgesic Anti-convulsant Anti-depressant Anti-diarrheal Anti-dystonia Anti-emetic Anti-inflammation Anti-microbial Anti-oxidant Anti-prion Anti-proliferative Anti-psychotic Anxiolytic Cardioprotective Cognitive protective Immune modulation Neuroprotection Somnolence	15, 16, 19–101

*Scientific references are located at the end of the book following the glossary, in numerical order.

(Continued)

TABLE 1. *(Continued)*

Cannabinoid	Abbreviation	Biological effects	Scientific Reference*
Cannabidiolic acid	CBDA	Anti-emetic Anti-proliferative	102–105
Cannabidivarin	CBDV	Anti-emetic Anti-convulsant	106–108
Cannabigerol	CBG	Anti-depressant Anti-inflammatory Anti-microbial Anti-proliferative	16, 20, 109–112
Cannabinol	CBN	Anti-coagulant Anti-diarrheal Anti-microbial	20, 113, 114
Δ9-tetrahydrocannabinol	THC	Addiction reduction Analgesic Anti-coagulant Anti-convulsant Anti-depressant Anti-dystonia Anti-emetic Anti-hypertensive Anti-inflammation Anti-oxidant Anti-microbial Anti-proliferative Anti-spasmodic Anti-tussive Anxiolytic Immune modulation Neuroprotection Orexigenic Somnolence	19, 21, 22, 36, 51, 56, 61, 68, 77, 79, 88, 89, 93, 94, 113–189
Δ9-tetrahydrocannabinolic acid	THCA	Anti-emetic Anti-nausea	102
Δ9-tetrahydrocannabivarin	THCV	Anti-emetic Anti-inflammation Neuroprotective Weight maintenance	108, 190–192

Routes of administration of cannabis/cannabinoids

Cannabis is prepared in its natural herbal form in various ways that are known by a variety of terms. It may be used as the seeded mixture of flowers, leaves, and stems; as the seedless unfertilized female flowering tops, known as "sensemilla" in North America; and as the resin collected from the flowers and commonly known as "hashish" or "hash" in North America. "Kif" is finely sifted cannabis that, in some regions of the world, are mixed with tobacco.[193] The terms described here are all found throughout the literature, but you should be aware that there is quite a bit of geographical, cultural, and generational variation in how these terms may be used, and other terms continue to be originated.

Russo[3] gives an excellent discussion of historical prescriptions and preparations of cannabis for medical purposes. A ninth century Persian concoction of herbs and juice from cannabis was administered to treat migraine and other types of pain, to prevent miscarriage, and, in large quantities, to prevent pregnancy. In tenth century Persia, cannabis leaves were apparently used to stimulate hair growth. In the nineteenth century it spread from India, where it was used to treat tetanus, to Britain and North America, where it was to be used as a muscle relaxer, antispasmodic, anti-migraine, analgesic, and even anti-depressant.

In modern times, smoking and oral ingestion are the most common methods of cannabis use. The United Patients Group website for alternative medicine (**www.unitedpatientsgroup.com**) provides an informative list of ways that medical cannabis can be consumed. These are briefly described here, and interested readers are referred to the website.

Smoking remains the most common method of cannabis consumption, and effects are noticed almost immediately. Marijuana can be smoked in a hand-rolled cigarette (a "joint"), in a tobacco cigar/cigarette that has been emptied and refilled with a mix of tobacco and cannabis (a "blunt"), in a pipe, or in a water pipe (a "bong"). Smoking is not a particularly healthy way to consume cannabis, as inhalation of combusted matter is typically irritating to the respiratory system, may introduce carcinogens, and can lead to increased risk of respiratory diseases and cancer.

A systematic review of the literature on the effectiveness of smoked cannabis for relief of chronic non-cancer pain[194] found that this might be of use for patients with severe neuropathic pain that has not responded to other standard treatments. Based on observational studies, they caution that cannabis should not be smoked by patients younger than 25 years of age, those who have current or past history or family history of psychosis, those who are pregnant or planning pregnancy, and those who have anxiety or mood disorders. More information about these conditions can be found in Chapters 3 and 4. Kahan and colleagues[194] also recommend a maximum dose of 1 inhalation 4 times per day (about 400 mg per day) of dried cannabis containing 9% THC. As research into cannabis as medicine continues, these dosage recommendations will likely change.

A newer alternative to smoking of cannabis is use of a vaporizer. Vaporizers heat up the plant at a temperature sufficient to allow release of the active components for inhalation, without reaching the point of combustion. It is thought that inhalation of vaporized cannabis may reduce some of the health hazards of smoking, while still offering the same benefits. The United Patients Group website offers helpful links for pre-purchase research on vaporizers.

Ingestion of cannabis has been suggested for pain relief, spasticity, and sleep disorders. The effects on the body occur more slowly and may be less likely to give a "high" feeling that is associated with smoking. United Patients Group warns that it is much easier to over-consume marijuana edibles because it takes longer to feel the effect, and because the edibles taste good (who doesn't love brownies?) Additionally, the website explains that eating raw cannabis is not recommended, but rather that cannabis edibles are made with butters or oils derived from the plant. Soaking leaves, stems, and buds of cannabis in boiling water can create a tea; it is suggested that alcohol, oil, or butter should be added to this tea in order to dissolve the THC. Apparently, some dispensaries even carry marijuana sodas!

Cannabis also comes in tinctures and tonics that can be added to foods and beverages, placed directly in the mouth, or applied to the skin. These methods are recommended for patients suffering nausea and vomiting associated with some medical conditions and as may occur when undergoing chemotherapy. Tinctures and tonics are made by soaking cannabis flowers and leaves in alcohol. Cannabis also can be made into balms, salves, lotions and ointments from cannabis oil, and can be rubbed directly onto the skin. United Patients Group suggests that these topical applications are free from psychoactive reactions, and can be very effective as analgesics and anti-inflammatories.

Another form of marijuana, hash, made from the resin of female cannabis flowers, is compressed into small blocks of a waxy substance. This can be eaten, smoked, and added to edibles and teas. Hash is reported to have a much higher concentration of THC than dried cannabis – the University of Washington Alcohol and Drug Abuse Institute (adai.uw.edu/marijuana/factsheets/potency.htm) indicates that the strongest THC concentration is found in hash oil, which may contain 15% to 30% THC, while hash can contain 10% to 20% THC. In comparison, the THC content of dried cannabis varies greatly, from around 1% up to 20%.

Known effects of cannabinoids on the body

Cells in our bodies have proteins on their surfaces that act as receptors. These receptors can bind and interact with substances that are important signaling molecules, called neurotransmitters – they allow the cells of the body to communicate through the nervous system. The nervous system is talked about in two components: the central nervous system, or CNS, which includes the brain, spinal cord, and nerves, and the peripheral nervous system, or PNS, which includes the nerves and ganglia (clusters of nerve cells) outside of the brain and spinal cord. Nerve cells are called neurons. Neurons process signals through electrical and chemical signals.

One important signaling system in the vertebrate body is the endogenous cannabinoid system, or the endocannabinoid system. This system operates via receptors known as cannabinoid 1 (CB_1) and cannabinoid 2 (CB_2) and small active molecules called endocannabinoids. These receptors are reviewed in detail by Giacoppo et al.[11] and by Guindon and Hohman[195] and are briefly summarized in greatly simplified form here. CB_1 receptors are found in the central nervous system, and mainly expressed in areas involved in movement, attention and complex cognitive functions, learning, memory, and emotions. They are also found in some organs and other tissues of the body. CB_2 receptors are mostly found in cells of the immune system and hematopoietic systems, but are also present to some degree in the brain as well. The CB_1 receptors are responsible for balancing the signals in the CNS, keeping it from being overstimulated or over-inhibited. The CB_2 receptors respond to damaging events in the body and can release molecules that inhibit inflammation. There are likely receptors other than CB_1 and CB_2 that have yet to be discovered and characterized.

Endocannabinoids are molecules that are made in the cell membrane and that bind and activate the cannabinoid receptors. They operate to maintain a stable environment in the body, to signal between different systems, and have functions such as regulation of food intake and modulation of the immune system. The endocannabinoid system is also responsible for controlling nociception, a signal to the brain or spinal cord that indicates potential damage and is usually perceived as pain.[195]

The cannabinoids found in cannabis are termed exocannabinoids (as opposed to endocannabinoids, those made by the body itself). Exocannabinoids are receiving increased attention for their beneficial actions on the body, including analgesic, anti-anxiety, anti-depressant, anti-inflammatory, anti-oxidant, anti-proliferative, anti-spasmodic, anti-seizure, anti-viral, appetitive, immunomodulatory, neuroprotective, and sedative effects. Exocannabinoids are proving particularly effective in management of chronic pain.[196] It has been suggested that in some cases, cannabis may relieve conditions such as migraine, fibromyalgia, and irritable bowel syndrome because of an underlying endocannabinoid deficiency.[197] A large epidemiologic study of non-smokers and cannabis smokers examined the effects of cannabis on serum C-reactive protein, which is produced by the liver and released into the blood following injury, infection, or other causes of inflammation. In this study, cannabis smoking appeared to mediate the levels of C-reactive protein, acting as an anti-inflammatory agent.[198]

Recent studies have found cannabinoids can directly affect cancers via several anti-proliferative (anti-tumor) properties: apoptosis (cell death), anti-angiogenesis (prevention of tumor vascularization), and anti-metastasis (See Tables 1 and 2 for references), and is also being extensively studied as a treatment for neurodegenerative diseases such as Alzheimer's disease, amyotrophic lateral sclerosis (ALS), cerebral ischemia, Huntington's disease, multiple sclerosis (MS), and Parkinson's disease. These diseases are characterized by gradual and progressive loss of neurons. Although each of these diseases has a different cause and progression, they have several commonalities: neuro-inflammation, oxidative stress, excitotoxicity, protein misfolding, mitochondrial dysfunction, and altered endocannabinoid signaling .[11] Cannabis and the cannabinoids may hold promise to help reduce symptoms and delay progression. The known effects of cannabis are summarized in Table 2, which is divided into beneficial and detrimental effects—note that some effects, for example immunomodulatory, are in both categories. Immune modulation can be both helpful and harmful, depending upon other factors. Also note that some studies find conflicting results on the same effect – for example, some studies find that cannabis has anti-depressant effects, while others find that it can act as a depressant. Again, various factors (i.e., cannabinoid content of the cannabis strain used in the study, administration route of the cannabis, other factors unique to the study participants, etc.) may explain these seemingly contradictory results, and this highlights the necessity of further medical research on cannabis. Both types of effects are described in more detail in the references provided, and in the sections on specific conditions in Chapters 3 and 4.

TABLE 2. Effects of cannabis on the body

Effect	Scientific Reference*
Beneficial	
Addiction reduction	8, 83, 148–150, 164, 199–203
Analgesic	39, 40, 77, 95, 96, 98, 145, 147, 151, 154, 165, 194, 204–242
Anti-asthmatic	243
Anti-bacterial	20
Anti-coagulant	113
Anti-convulsant	32, 36, 37, 42, 57, 106, 107, 135, 180, 186, 187, 244–248
Anti-depressant	99, 117, 174, 249–251

*Scientific references are located at the end of the book following the glossary, in numerical order.

(Continued)

TABLE 2. *(Continued)*

Effect	Scientific Reference*
Anti-diarrheal	18, 31, 114, 238, 252
Anti-dystonia	38, 253
Anti-emetic	60, 79, 85, 102, 103, 108, 120, 128–130, 132–134, 136, 140, 153, 156, 157, 161, 166, 168–170, 179, 182, 183, 254–262
Anti-hypertensive	121, 131, 137, 181, 189, 263–267
Anti-inflammatory	17, 25, 28, 39, 40, 44, 56, 67, 71, 72, 78, 81, 111, 112, 127, 141, 159, 252, 268
Anti-oxidant	22, 27, 61, 81, 212
Anti-proliferative	16, 27, 51, 64, 68, 70, 82, 87, 89, 91, 94, 96, 104, 105, 110–112, 122–126, 142, 143, 146, 155, 158, 160, 172, 173, 175, 185, 188, 269–275
Anti-psychotic	47, 48, 55, 62, 63, 65, 74, 75, 84, 100, 101
Anti-spasmodic	171, 184, 210, 216, 232, 249, 276–285
Anti-tussive	159
Anti-viral	163, 286
Anxiolytic	26, 29, 30, 41, 53, 65, 73, 92, 139, 144, 220, 287, 288
Cardio-protective	49, 289
Cognitive protection	52, 66, 290
Immunomodulatory	28, 45, 46, 50, 54, 58, 59, 67, 71, 72, 76, 93, 97, 198, 286, 291–293
Neuroprotective	15, 22, 24, 25, 35, 43, 61, 69, 80, 90, 95, 96, 138, 191, 212, 294–300
Orexigenic	174, 178, 249, 301–307
Somnolence	33, 34, 167, 206, 207, 210, 220, 227, 232, 239, 240, 304, 305, 307
Weight maintenance	308–313
Detrimental	
Adipogenic	314, 315
Anxiogenic	131, 261, 316–333

*Scientific references are located at the end of the book following the glossary, in numerical order.

(Continued)

TABLE 2. *(Continued)*

Effect	Scientific Reference*
Carcinogenic	334–343
Cognitive impairment	344–347
Depressant	237, 261, 319, 332, 348–357
Emetic	261, 358–363
Hepatic alteration	364–368
Hyperalgesic	369
Hypertension	370
Hypotension	261
Immunomodulatory	93, 371–374
Insulin resistance	315
Neuroimpairment	375–387
Mania inducement	333, 388–394
Nystagmus inducement	395
Opioid dependence relapse	396–398
Pancreatitis	399–403
Perception alteration	261
Pro-convulsive	404–408
Pro-psychotic	261, 333, 409–463
Respiratory impairment	464–470
Stroke	405
Tachycardia	471
Vasoconstriction	472

CHAPTER 3

STATE-AUTHORIZED CONDITIONS AND THE EFFECTS OF CANNABIS ON THEM

Descriptions of conditions are summarized from the United States Centers for Disease Control (US CDC) **www.cdc.gov**, the World Health Organization (WHO) **www.who.int**, or the United States National Institutes of Health (NIH) **www.nih.gov** wherever possible. For some conditions, there are also private foundations with websites that have been referred to. Descriptions of the known beneficial effects of cannabis for these medical conditions are summarized from the scientific studies compiled in this guide. Following each description is a list of additional resources for that condition and the associated website address.

Table 3 presents the medical cannabis websites for each state as of time of this publication. These web addresses are presented here so that patients, physicians, caregiv-ers, growers, and dispensaries can find additional and up-to-date information for their states. Table 4 presents the state-approved conditions for which medical marijuana may be used, the known effects of cannabis on that condition (categorized as beneficial, no significant change and/or negative evaluation, and detrimental), and the scientific reference numbers for those effects. The corresponding scientific reference can be located at the end of the book, after the glossary, in numerical order.

TABLE 3. Internet addresses of state medical marijuana programs

Alaska	Alaska Department of Health and Social Services, Division of Public Health dhss.alaska.gov/dph/vitalstats/pages/marijuana.aspx
Arizona	Arizona Department of Health Services **www.azdhs.gov/medicalmarijuana**
California	California Department of Public Health **www.cdph.ca.gov/programs/mmp**
Colorado	Department of Public Health and Environment **www.colorado.gov/pacific/cdphe/medicalmarijuana**
Connecticut	Connecticut Department of Consumer Protection **www.ct.gov/dcp/cwp**
Delaware	Delaware Health and Social Services, Division of Public Health dhss.delaware.gov/dph/hsp/medmarhome.html
District of Columbia	Government of the District of Columbia Department of Health doh.dc.gov/service/medical-marijuana-program
Hawaii	State of Hawaii, Department of Health, STD/AIDS Prevention Branch health.hawaii.gov/std-aids/medical-marijuana-program
Illinois	Illinois Department of Public Health **www.idph.state.il.us/HealthWellness/MedicalCannabis**
Maine	Maine Department of Health and Human Services **www.maine.gov/dhhs/dlrs/mmm**
Maryland	Maryland Medical Marijuana Commission mmc.maryland.gov
Massachusetts	Massachusetts Health and Human Services Departments and Divisions **www.mass.gov/eohhs/gov/departments/dph/programs/hcq/medical-marijuana**
Michigan	Michigan Department of Licensing and Regulatory Affairs **www.michigan.gov/lara**
Minnesota	Minnesota Department of Health **www.health.state.mn.us/topics/cannabis**
Montana	Montana Department of Health and Human Services **www.Dphhs.mt.gov**
Nevada	Nevada Division of Public and Behavioral Health **http://www.health.nv.gov/MedicalMarijuana.htm**
New Hampshire	New Hampshire Department of Health and Human Services **www.dhhs.state.nh.us/oos/tcp**
New Jersey	State of New Jersey Department of Health **www.state.nj.us/health/medicalmarijuana**
New Mexico	New Mexico Department of Health nmhealth.org/about/mcp/svcs
New York	New York State Medical Marijuana Program **www.health.ny.gov/regulations/medical_marijuana**

(Continued)

TABLE 3. *(Continued)*

Oregon	Oregon Public Health Division public.health.oregon.gov/diseasesconditions/chronicdisease/medicalmarijuanaprogram
Rhode Island	State of Rhode Island Department of Health **www.health.ri.gov/healthcare/medicalmarijuana**
Vermont	Vermont Crime Information Center vcic.vermont.gov.marijuana_registry
Washington	Washington State Department of Health **www.doh.wa.gov/youandyourfamily/marijuana/medicalmarijuanacannabis**

Acquired Immune Deficiency Syndrome (AIDS) (see also HIV)

AIDS is a suite of symptoms and/or infections resulting from the deterioration of the immune system due to infection with the HIV virus. The HIV, or Human Immunodeficiency Virus, is transmitted through bodily fluids (blood, penile, vaginal and rectal fluids, and breast milk). Viruses are parasitic on their host cells (the host is the organism that the virus infects, in this case, the human) and rely upon them to reproduce themselves and infect other cells in the host's body, and then to be passed on to other hosts. HIV predominantly infects a person's T-helper (CD4) immune cells. Because HIV kills the important immune cells that it infects, the person becomes more vulnerable to infections, even those that individuals with healthy immune systems can resist. AIDS.gov lists more than twenty common opportunistic infections considered "AIDS-defining conditions". Among them are certain fungal infections, bacterial infections including tuberculosis, and viral infections. There is currently no known cure for AIDS. It is important to know that not everyone who is infected with HIV will develop AIDS. Research and development of antiretroviral drugs have made it possible for the virus to be controlled in a person's body. Typically a person must take a combination of medications rather than just one. The medications do have debilitating side effects however, and some are severe. More information on side effects of HIV/AIDS medications and the benefits of cannabis can be found in the section on Treatment with AZT, chemotherapy, protease inhibitors, and radiotherapy in this chapter.

Cannabis helps relieve many of the symptoms of AIDS such as nausea, appetite loss, depression, and pain.[304, 474, 475, 478] Two clinical trials [205, 218] found that herbal cannabis significantly relieved otherwise intractable HIV neuropathy. Studies of simian immunodeficiency virus (SIV) in laboratory nonhuman primates found that THC administered before and during infection slowed disease progression, reduced viral load and tissue inflammation, and overall reduced morbidity and mortality.[291, 292] Cannabinoids help decrease the amount of the virus, reduce inflammation, and slow progression of AIDS by modulating the host's immune system.[286, 473, 659] Additionally, cannabis component denbinobin was found in a laboratory study to directly affect the HIV virus, prohibiting it from effectively replicating itself in host cells.[119] While cannabis has beneficial antiviral properties in a developed organism, it is important to note that data from animal studies indicate that exposure of the developing fetus to cannabis could detrimentally alter the immune system and, among other effects, reduce the immune response to viruses.[481]

Additional AIDS resources:
AIDS 2014: www.aids2014.org
AIDS.gov: www.aids.gov
AIDS.org: www.aids.org
AVERT: www.avert.org
UNAIDS: www.unaids.org
US Centers for Disease Control:
www.cdc.gov
World Health Organization:
www.who.int

Alzheimer's disease

Alzheimer's disease is a progressive form of dementia characterized by memory loss. It occurs when abnormal proteins accumulate in the brain and form deposits called "amyloid plaques" and "tau tangles", which cause nerve cells to begin to function less efficiently, hindering communication between them. According to the National Institute on Aging, this degenerative process probably begins at least a decade before symptoms are evident. As damage spreads throughout the brain, the portion that forms memories (the "hippocampus") becomes damaged and memory loss begins. By the final stages of Alzheimer's disease, the brain has shrunk considerably because of widespread plaque and tangle formation.

Alzheimer's disease is most common in people over 60 years of age, and impairs a person's ability to converse, respond to the environment, and carry out daily activities. Ultimately, in the final stages of the disease the patient cannot communicate and is completely bedridden. The US CDC reports that in 2013 there were some 5 million Americans with Alzheimer's disease. There is currently no known cure.

Cannabis has neuroprotective effects that continue to be studied for their therapeutic potential in neurodegenerative diseases. In mouse models of Alzheimer's disease, CBD was shown to suppress formation of amyloid plaques[44] and to have beneficial effects on learning behavior.[69] Both THC and CBD have antioxidant properties[22] that may preserve cell integrity and help slow the progression of neurodegeneration,[90, 138, 482, 484] thereby aiding in the preservation of memory.

Additional Alzheimer's disease resources:
Alzheimer's Association: www.alz.org
Alzheimer Europe:
www.alzheimer-europe.org
Alzheimer's Foundation of America:
www.alzfdn.org
Alzforum: www.alzforum.org
Alzheimers.gov: www.alzheimers.gov
Brightfocus Foundation:
www.brightfocus.org/alzheimers
Fisher Center for Alzheimer's Research Foundation: www.alzinfo.org
National Institute on Aging:
www.nia.nih.gov

Amyotrophic Lateral Sclerosis (ALS)

Amyotrophic lateral sclerosis (ALS) is a progressive neurological disease that affects voluntary movement. It is also known as Lou Gehrig's disease, after a famous early twentieth century baseball player who contracted and died from ALS. Ultimately, death of nerve cells in the brain and spinal cord cause loss of movement of muscles throughout the body. Only the nerves that affect voluntary movements are affected by ALS, and thus the heart and digestive system are not directly involved in ALS. Early symptoms of ALS are weakness of arms and legs, and difficulty speaking, swallowing, and breathing – ultimately, weakening and atrophy of muscles leads to paralysis and death. Average survival with ALS is three to five years, but there are also people, such as Stephen Hawking, who have lived with the disease for more than ten years. The cause of ALS is unknown, although up to 10% of cases occur within families, and at least two genetic mutations have been identified that are present in a significant number of ALS patients. There may also be environmental factors involved in non-familial cases of the disease. The National Institute of Neurological Disorders and Stroke reports that the disease is most commonly diagnosed between ages 60 and 69, and that more than 12,000 Americans are living with ALS. There is currently no known cure.

Cannabis has neuroprotective effects that continue to be studied for their therapeutic potential in neurodegenerative diseases. Studies in mice indicate that Cannabis has antioxidative, anti-inflammatory and neuroprotective[294] effects that may help slow the progression of ALS[300,486] via the cannabinoid receptors.[488] In addition, marijuana helps to reduce symptoms of pain, anxiety, anorexia, depression, spasticity, drooling and sleep disturbances[249]. Research into medical cannabis for ALS may hold the keys to improvement of quality of life and even reduction in the course and severity of the disease.[485,487]

Additional ALS resources:
ALS Therapy Development Institute: www.als.net
American Speech-Language-Hearing Association: www.asha.org
The ALS Association: www.alsa.org
Muscular Dystrophy Association: mda.org
National Institute of Neurological Disorders and Stroke:
www.ninds.nih.gov
World Federation of Neurology Research Group on Motor Neuron
Diseases: www.wfnals.org

Anorexia

Anorexia is defined as a prolonged lack of appetite. Anorexia may be caused by medical conditions or treatments for such that cause a person to lose appetite. A specific condition, anorexia nervosa, is an eating disorder characterized by refusal to eat so as to lose weight or avoid weight gain. Anorexia can have serious consequences, including deterioration of several organ systems. In an experimental study on laboratory rats, cannabis positively stimulated energy intake, and in a dose-response manner (meaning the more cannabis, the more energy intake).[306] In humans with debilitating conditions such as Hepatitis C virus infection,[489] human immunodeficiency virus infection,[493] inflammatory bowel disease,[490] and multiple sclerosis,[491] cannabis has moderate to strong orexigenic (appetite stimulation) effects.[301, 302, 492]

Arnold-Chiari malformation

Arnold-Chiari malformation is structural defect in the part of the brain that controls balance. In this condition, the cerebellum is pushed downward into the foramen magnum (the opening through which the spinal cord attaches to the brain) and into the upper spinal canal. The National Institute of Neurological Disorders and Stroke indicates that Arnold-Chiari malformations are classified into 4 or 5 types, depending upon how severe the disorder is and what parts of the brain intrude on the spinal cord. Arnold-Chiari malformation can be caused by defects that occur during fetal development from genetic mutations or lack of certain nutrients, or later in life due to injury, exposure to harmful substances, or infection. Symptoms of Arnold-Chiari malformation are neck pain, balance issues and dizziness, muscle weakness, numbness of extremities, vision and hearing issues, insomnia, depression, nausea and vomiting, and severe headaches. Treatments include medications for symptoms, and sometimes surgery for more serious types.

Cannabis has analgesic, anti-nausea, and anti-emetic effects that may be useful to treat symptoms. See references for Migraine; Pain: chronic/intractable/severe; Nausea; Vomiting: intractable.

Additional Arnold-Chiari malformation resources:
American Syringomyelia Alliance Project Inc: asap.org
Conquer Chiari:
www.conquerchiari.org
National Institute of Neurological Disorders and Stroke:
www.ninds.nih.gov
National Organization for Rare Disorders: www.rarediseases.org
Spina Bifida Association: www.spinabifidaassociation.org
The Chiari Institute:
www.chiariinstitute.com
The World Arnold Chiari Malformation Association: www.wacma.com

Arthritis

Arthritis comprises more than 100 diseases and conditions that affect the joints and their surrounding and connective tissues – these are also known as "rheumatic diseases." Arthritis causes inflammation and pain, and is reported by the US CDC to affect 1 in 5 US adults. Arthritis can be caused by trauma, infection, or autoimmune conditions—rheumatoid arthritis is believed to be caused by the immune system and affects multiple joints throughout the body. The US CDC categorizes six common forms of arthritis: childhood arthritis, fibromyalgia, gout, osteoarthritis, rheumatoid arthritis, and systemic lupus erythematosus (SLE or lupus). We also include a less common, but debilitating form of arthritis, called ankylosing spondylitis.

- *Childhood Arthritis* is broadly defined as occurring in people younger than 16 years of age. Childhood arthritis comprises many different types of arthritis, typically classified into juvenile rheumatoid arthritis (JRA), juvenile chronic arthritis (JCA), and juvenile idiopathic arthritis (JIA), although other forms also exist. JRA is the most common arthritis in children, with three subtypes. Systemic JRA is a severe form that may affect many body systems in addition to the joints. The peak age of onset is 1 to 6 years of age. Polyarticular JRA affects five or more joints, and is more common in females. Pauciarticular JRA (also known as oligoarticular) affects fewer than five joints, and is also more common in females. The CDC estimated that in 2007 there were 294,000 children in the United States with arthritis conditions that can severely impact the quality of life.

- *Fibromyalgia* is a debilitating disorder of as yet unknown cause, although it may be associated with stressful or traumatic events, repetitive injuries, infectious or autoimmune disease, obesity, or genetic predisposition. Patients experience widespread pain in the absence of another disorder that would explain it, fatigue and sleep disturbances, and psychological distress. The disorder may co-occur with rheumatoid arthritis, systemic lupus erythematosus, or ankylosing spondylitis. Common symptoms of fibromyalgia are morning stiffness and tingling or numbness of extremities, headaches and migraines, irritable bowel syndrome, and what is known as "fibro fog" (problems with thinking and memory). The CDC estimates that approximately 5 million adults were affected with fibromyalgia in 2005, with approximately a 7:1 female to male ratio. Prevalence of the disease increases with age, and it is usually diagnosed in middle age, although children can also be affected. Fibromyalgia negatively impacts quality of life, and adults with the disorder average almost 3 times as many missed days of work as adults without fibromyalgia.

- *Gout* is an extremely painful inflammatory arthritis that results from uric acid crystal deposition in tissues and fluids caused by too much uric acid in the blood. The condition can be caused by some medications, alcohol, or a diet rich in meat and seafood, and is associated with excess weight, hypertension, and an increased risk for kidney stones. There are progressive stages of gout, including acute flare-ups that can last days to weeks, with mild to severe pain. The great toe is most commonly affected. Gout is more often seen in men than women, and the CDC reports that approximately 6.1 million US adults were affected in 2005. Treatments for gout include anti-inflammatory drugs, steroids, colchicine, dietary changes, weight loss, and management of other medications that may contribute to excess blood uric acid.

- *Osteoarthritis* (OA) is also known as degenerative joint disease. Breakdown of the cartilage and other tissues of the joint results from a variety of causes, is usually gradual, and the damage is cumulative over time. The most commonly affected joints are in the knees, hips, hands, and spine. There is currently no cure for OA, and treatment focuses on managing pain and improving joint function. Healthy weight maintenance can help relieve symptoms and slow the progression of joint deterioration, medications can be prescribed for pain, and physical and occupational therapy can help manage the symptoms. Treatments for more extensive OA can include cortisone shots into the joint, injections of lubricating fluids, and joint replacement surgery. The US CDC estimates that in 2005, 33.6% (12.4 million) of US adults age 65 or older were affected by OA. Osteoarthritis can severely impact the quality of life, and some 80% of osteoarthritis sufferers have limited movement—according to the CDC, 25% of patients cannot perform major activities of daily living.

- *Rheumatoid arthritis* (RA) is an autoimmune condition in which a chronic inflammatory process causes damage to the lining of 5 or more joints, and other organ systems may also be affected. RA is more common in women than in men, and onset typically occurs in the sixties, although people of any age can be affected (see juvenile rheumatoid arthritis). The CDC estimates that in 2005, 0.6% (1.5 million) of US adults age 18 or over were affected by RA. Rheumatoid arthritis severely impacts quality of life, even more than does osteoarthritis. Although RA affects a relatively low percentage of Americans, it accounts for a high proportion of disability cases. There is no cure for RA, but if the disease is diagnosed within 6 months of the onset of symptoms, early and aggressive treatment may facilitate remission of the disease within 5 years of diagnosis. For people with polycyclic or progressive RA, treatment includes anti-inflammatory and anti-rheumatic medications, and physical and occupational therapy.

- *Systemic lupus erythematosus* (SLE) is an autoimmune disease of unknown cause, although it is associated with genetic, environmental, and hormonal conditions. SLE is characterized by widespread inflammation and tissue damage, including to the joints. Symptoms include fatigue, joint pain and swelling, fevers, and skin rashes. Females are much more likely to have SLE than males, and people of African origin are more likely to be affected than those of European origin. The

US CDC reports that SLE can occur at any age, but is most common between ages 15 and 40. Because SLE can be difficult to diagnose, it is difficult to estimate the number of people affected, and CDC cites studies that estimate anywhere from 161,000 to 1,500,000 cases. There is no cure for SLE, but treatment includes immunosuppressive and corticosteroid medications. These medications can have serious side effects, and treatment compliance can be an issue.

- *Ankylosing spondylitis* primarily affects the spine. According to the Spondylitis Association of America, inflammation of the vertebrae leads to severe, chronic pain. When ankylosing spondylitis is advanced, new bone forms on the spine until it is fused, leading to immobility and a forward-stooped posture. The area where the sacrum (at the bottom of the vertebral column) meets the pelvis is typically involved. Inflammation, pain, and stiffness of other parts of the body are also common.. A genetic variant has been found that is associated with ankylosing spondylitis, but it is thought that environmental factors such as a bacterial infection may ultimately trigger the disease. Ankylosing spondylitis is characterized by episodes known as "flares", in which inflammation, immobility, fatigue and pain are pronounced and accompanied by emotional symptoms of depression, withdrawal, and anger. Brophy and Calin[501] questioned 214 ankylosing spondylitis patients to characterize flare, and additionally found that relief from the symptoms of flare can be obtained in some cases by cannabis.

The cannabinoids have strong anti-inflammatory properties, and can be beneficial against arthritis directly, as well as indirectly, to relieve symptoms. In a mouse model of arthritis, cannabidiol blocked progression of disease processes.[67] In a human study of rheumatoid arthritis, orally-administered cannabis[208] was associated with a significant reduction in disease. Several studies also report that cannabis significantly reduces pain and helps improve mood. A Cochrane systematic review conducted by Lynch and Campbell[229] included 18 clinical trials of cannabinoids to treat chronic, non-cancer pain, including a study of fibromyalgia and one of rheumatoid arthritis. Cannabinoids helped to relieve pain, improve function, and improve sleep. Side effects were mild to moderate and well tolerated. A clinical trial of THC administered to fibromyalgia patients in Germany found that, in the absence of other pain medication, some patients experienced a significant reduction in pain.[536]

Additional Arthritis resources:
American Academy of Orthopedic Surgeons: orthoinfo.aaos.org
American College of Rheumatology: www.rheumatology.org
American Podiatric Medical Association: www.apma.org
Arthritis Foundation: www.arthritis.org
Fibromyalgia Network: www.fmnetnews.com
National Fibromyalgia Association: www.fmaware.org
National Fibromyalgia & Chronic Pain Association: www.fmpcaware.org
National Institute of Arthritis and Musculoskeletal and Skin Diseases: www.niams.nih.gov
National Library of Medicine: www.ncbi.nlm.nih.gov
S.L.E. Lupus Foundation: www.lupusny.org
Spondylitis Association of America: www.spondylitis.org
The American Fibromyalgia Syndrome Association, Inc.: www.afsafund.org
The Arthritis Society of Canada: www.arthritis.ca
US Centers for Disease Control and Prevention: www.cdc.gov

Cachexia

Cachexia is a wasting syndrome associated with chronic illnesses such as cancer, AIDS, diabetes, and multiple sclerosis. Muscle mass and adipose tissue (fat) diminish, and the patient suffers severe weight loss. Cachexia can ultimately lead to immobility due to muscle loss. A recent review article of cancer cachexia[660] considers the condition a preventable comorbidity (a disorder that occurs with the primary disease) of cancer that is associated with decreased response to therapy and poor prognosis. Although research advances have helped elucidate the causes of cachexia, insufficient attention has been given to the nutritional and metabolic changes that go along with cancer and other cachexia causing conditions. The appetite stimulating effects of cannabis have been known for years.[303, 516, 517] A study of CB1 receptors in rats indicated that administration of the endocannabinoid anandamide (which is chemically similar to THC) stimulated these receptors and resulted in increased food consumption.[518] In laboratory mice, THC stimulated the CB1 receptors at doses that did not affect motor skills, and increased food consumption in a dose-dependent manner (meaning that the more THC, the more food consumed).[118]

Cancer

Cancers are diseases in which cells lose the normal regulation on growth and divide without control. Cancerous cells multiply, and in most cases cause a mass, called a "tumor". Not all tumors are cancers, but tumors that spread to other areas of the body are cancerous. Cancerous cells multiply and can invade other tissues, both local and throughout the body—the process of a cancer spreading to a different region is called "metastasis." A cancer is usually named for the location of its origin – lung cancer began in the lung, for example, although it may ultimately metastasize to other organs. The National Cancer Institute reports that there are more than 100 different types of cancer.

There are a large number of treatments available for cancers, and typically more than one is used. The most common treatment methods are chemotherapies, which use drugs to slow or stop the growth of cancerous cells, radiation therapy to kill the cancerous cells, and immunotherapies that help the body's own immune system fight against cancerous cells. Chemotherapy and radiotherapy are known for the negative side effects that they cause, and marijuana has been found to be particularly effective at easing some of these. The National Cancer Institute lists the side effects of anemia, excessive bleeding, appetite changes, nausea, vomiting, difficulty with digestion, urination, and defecation, fatigue, hair loss, infection, memory loss, changes to the mouth, throat, skin, peripheral neuropathy (nerve problems), pain and swelling, hearing and movement problems, and sexual and fertility problems.

Recent studies have found cannabinoids can directly affect cancers via several anti-tumoral properties: apoptosis (cell death), anti-angiogenesis (prevention of tumor vascularization), and anti-metastasis.[16, 27, 51, 54, 64, 68, 70, 82, 87, 91, 94, 104, 105, 110, 112, 122–126, 142, 143, 146, 155, 158, 160, 172, 175, 185, 188, 217, 269–272, 274, 275, 313, 334, 502–511] A recent study of prostate cancer cells found that there are substantially more CB1 and CB2 receptors found on cancer cells than non-cancer cells. Treating the cancer cells with endocannabinoids caused apoptosis – thus, cannabinoids may act on the CB1 and CB2 receptors of cancer cells in a similar way to endocannabinoids.[661] Cannabinoids have been shown to help activate the cellular defenses against cancer to inhibit tumor growth,[158, 274] shrink tumors,[510] and inhibit cancer cell migration.[82, 104] Recently, Scott and colleagues[89] showed that cannabis compounds administered prior to radiation therapy help to drastically shrink tumors from a deadly form of brain cancer. In a cohort study of over 84,000 men, cannabis use was significantly associated with a 45% reduction in bladder cancer incidence.[512] Marijuana also benefits cancer patients indirectly by easing medical side effects such as pain, anxiety, nausea and anorexia (see entries for these conditions).

Additional Cancer resources:
American Cancer Society: www.cancer.org
Cancer Research Institute: www.cancerresearch.org
Cancer Research UK: www.cancerresearchuk.org
Cancer Treatment Centers of America: www.cancercenter.com
Cancer.Net: www.cancer.net
CancerCare: www.cancercare.org
National Cancer Institute: www.cancer.gov
US Centers for Disease Control and Prevention: www.cdc.gov
World Health Organization: www.who.int

Chronic inflammatory demyelinating polyneuropathy (CIPD)

CIPD is a neurological disorder that is also known as chronic relapsing polyneuropathy. It is characterized by progressive weakness and altered sensory function in the limbs. CIPD is caused by damage to the myelin sheath of the peripheral nerves, and can occur at any age. The National Institute of Neurological Disorders and Stroke indicates that it is more common in young adults and in males. Symptoms include tingling or numbness in extremities, weakness of limbs, loss of deep tendon reflexes, fatigue, and abnormal sensations. Treatments include corticosteroids and immunosuppressant drugs, and physical therapy. The prognosis of the disease varies widely, with some people having spontaneous recovery and others having episodes of partial recovery and relapses.

Cannabis has known anti-inflammatory, immunomodulatory, and analgesic properties that can benefit people with neuropathies. See the section on Peripheral neuropathy for more information and references.

Additional Chronic inflammatory demyelinating polyneuropathy resources:
GBS/CIDP Foundation International: www.gbs-cipd.org
National Institute of Neurological Disorders and Stroke: www.ninds.nih.gov

Chronic renal failure

Chronic renal failure is also known as chronic kidney disease. Kidneys are responsible for filtering the blood, and when they become damaged, waste remains in the body. Over time, damaged kidneys may fail altogether, and either regular dialysis or a kidney transplant is necessary. The US CDC estimates that more than 10% of US adults have varying degrees of chronic kidney disease. Risk for developing chronic kidney disease increases after age 50, and the most common risk factors include diabetes, high blood pressure, obesity, high cholesterol, and lupus. Kidneys can also be damaged by infections, drugs, or toxins. Management of risk factors is the most effective treatment. A study of cannabis compound cannabidiol in rats showed that it attenuated kidney damage via its antioxidant and anti-inflammatory properties[46].

Additional Chronic renal failure resources:
National Kidney Foundation:
www.kidney.org
US Centers for Disease Control and Prevention: www.cdc.gov

Cirrhosis

Cirrhosis refers to damage of the liver. Common causes are chronic alcohol abuse, fat deposition, cystic fibrosis, autoimmune conditions, and infections from macroparasites or viruses such as hepatitis B (HBV) or hepatitis C (HCV). These conditions cause injuries that scar the liver during its healing processes. If scarring is.advanced, the liver ceases to function properly and symptoms such as fatigue, jaundice, nausea and loss of appetite, weight loss, and bleeding problems may occur. If cirrhosis is not yet advanced, treatment to control the underlying cause (such as alcohol cessation or medications to control infections) can help slow the progression. The cannabis compound cannabidiol reduces inflammation in the liver, and has been shown to cause destruction of cells that exacerbate scarring[519]. Animal models of liver damage showed that cannabidiol prevented inflammation and further injury,[15] even independent of the cannabinoid receptors.[76] Cannabis also helps stimulate appetite, control nausea, and alleviate pain (see also Anorexia; Nausea; Pain: chronic/severe/intractable).

Additional Cirrhosis resources:
American Gastroenterological Association: www.gastro.org
American Liver Foundation: www.liverfoundation.org
PBCers Organization: pbcers.org

Crohn's disease (see also Inflammatory bowel disease)

Crohn's disease is a type of inflammatory bowel disease that affects the entire digestive tract. Typically there can be patches of diseased bowel with normal healthy tissue in between. The causes of Crohn's disease are not yet known, although an abnormal immune response to the harmless intestinal bacteria is involved. The US CDC and the Crohn's & Colitis Foundation of America report that Crohn's disease affects about 700,000 Americans, and is commonly diagnosed between the ages of 15 and 35. Common symptoms are diarrhea, abdominal cramps and pain, fever, rectal bleeding, loss of appetite, weight loss, and fatigue. Serious complications can occur, including intestinal blockage, sores or ulcers, and increased risk of colon cancer. Treatments include medications to help suppress the immune inflammatory response, care and attention to diet, and surgery to remove damaged sections of bowel. These treatments will not cure the disease, and relapse is common throughout life. Surveys of patients with ulcerative colitis and Crohn's disease indicate that cannabis is commonly used to reduce chronic pain and symptoms,[523] and although there is an association with higher risk of surgery,[238] it is not clear if this is caused by the cannabis, or quite likely due to greater need to alleviate symptoms in patients with more severe disease. In an observational study,[521] cannabis administered to Crohn's disease patients reduced disease activity and need for other medications and surgery. In patients whose disease did not respond to conventional medications, THC reduced symptoms, increased appetite, and improved sleep.[307] It is thought that at least part of the efficacy of cannabis to treat Crohn's disease is due to its action on the cannabinoid receptors.[522]

Additional Crohn's disease resources:
American Gastroenterological Association: www.gastro.org
Crohn's & Colitis:
www.crohnsandcolitisinfo.com
Crohn's & Colitis Foundation of America: www.cfa.org
Crohn's & Me: www.crohnsandme.com
National Institute of Diabetes and Digestive and Kidney Diseases:
www.niddk.nih.gov
US Centers for Disease Control and Prevention: www.cdc.gov

Dystonias

Dystonias are movement disorders in which involuntary muscle contractions cause repetitive movements, tremors, or abnormal postures. Cervical dystonia is also known as "spasmodic torticollis" or "torticollis." The National Institute of Neurological Disorders and Stroke indicates that cervical dystonia is the most common of the dystonias that are localized to a specific body part. It can occur at any age, although it is most commonly identified in middle age. The cause of dystonia is not currently known. There is no known cure, and no medications to slow the progression of dystonia or prevent it. There are treatments to alleviate symptoms of cervical dystonia, including botulinum toxin, various medications, deep brain stimulation, surgeries, and physical therapy. Cannabis can help to relieve pain and spasms[38] associated with dystonia, and has been reported to provide a significant level of clinical improvement in at least three cases.[152, 253, 526]

Additional Dystonia resources:
American Dystonia Society: www.dystoniasociety.org
Dystonia Europe: dystonia-europe.org
Global Dystonia Registry: www.globaldytstoniaregistry.org
Medical Research Foundation: www.dystonia-foundation.org
National Health Service: www.nhs.uk
National Institute of Neurological Disorders and Stroke: www.ninds.nih.gov
National Organization for Rare Diseases: www.rarediseases.org
Rare Diseases Clinical Research Network: www.rarediseasesnetwork.org
ST Dystonia: www.spasmodictorticollis.org
The Bachmann-Strauss Dystonia & Parkinson Foundation, Inc.: www.dystonia-parkinsons.org
The Dystonia Society: www.dystonia.org.uk
The Movement Disorder Society: www.movementdisorders.org
Tyler's Hope for a Dystonia Cure: www.tylershope.org

Epilepsy

Epilepsy is a neurological disorder that is characterized by seizures. The US CDC reports that 2.3 million adults and 450,000children in the United States have epilepsy. There are different types of seizures and different causes of seizures. Known causes of epilepsy include stroke, brain tumor, central nervous system infection, Alzheimer's disease and head/traumatic brain injury, but people can also develop epilepsy with none of these conditions. Seizures impair quality of life in a number of ways for epilepsy patients, and can be developmentally damaging in children. Dravet's Syndrome is a rare form of epilepsy that begins in infancy and lasts throughout life. The Epilepsy Foundation (www.epilepsy.com) reports that a known genetic mutation is responsible for about 80% of cases of Dravet's Syndrome. It is particularly difficult to treat because the seizures do not respond well to anti-convulsant medications.

The anti-convulsive effects of smoked cannabis have been known since the 1970s[244], and these effects were verified in several different animal models.[32, 36, 37, 106, 107, 135, 180, 186, 187, 245, 634] Cannabinoids are receiving increased attention as a therapy for epilepsy,[42, 246, 248, 529, 531, 631, 633] particularly in children.[527] A survey of parents who administered CBD-enriched marijuana to their children who had treatment-resistant epilepsies found that seizure frequency was reduced following cannabis.[532] Further, children were reported to have increased alertness, better moods, and sleep improvement, with minimal side effects of drowsiness and fatigue. In a case reported in the journal *Epilepsia*,[247] Charlotte Figi, a child with Dravet's Syndrome, was treated with a special strain of cannabis now known as "Charlotte's Web." Charlotte's epilepsy was refractory to treatment, and by age 5 the little girl suffered up to 50 seizures per day, had delayed cognition and motor skills, and required a feeding tube. Charlotte's physician began administering low doses of a preparation made from a high-CBD strain of marijuana, and slowly increased the dose while decreasing her other anti-convulsive medications. Eventually her other medications were discontinued, and after 20 months of cannabis treatment, Charlotte's seizures were reported to have been reduced to 2-3 per month. The child was able to eat and drink on her own, she began sleeping through the night, and she began walking and talking on her own.

Additional Epilepsy resources:
American Epilepsy Society: www.aesnet.org
CURE Epilepsy: www.cureepilepsy.org
Epilepsy Advocate: www.epilepsyadvocate.com
International Epilepsy Day: www.epilepsy.org
The Epilepsy Foundation: www.epilepsy.com
National Institute of Neurological Disorders and Stroke:
www.ninds.nih.gov
US Centers for Disease Control and Prevention: www.cdc.gov
World Health Organization: www.who.int

Fibromyalgia (see Arthritis)

Fibrous Dysplasia

Fibrous dysplasia is an uncommon disorder of the skeleton in which too much connective tissue is formed, and healthy bone is replaced with the fibrous connective tissue. Any bone in the body can be affected, but the National Institute of Arthritis and Musculoskeletal and Skin Diseases reports that the most commonly affected bones are the skull and face, femur (thigh bone), tibia (shin bone), humerus (upper arm bone), pelvis, and ribs. One or multiple bones can be affected. The disorder is thought to occur early in fetal development, and although it is caused by a defective gene, it is not inherited from parents and cannot be passed on to an affected person's children. Symptoms are painful, misshapen, and/or broken bones. People with affected skull or face bones may have the shape of those bones changed, and rarely may also have hearing or vision loss. Fibrous dysplasia has no cure, and treatment involves caring for symptoms, medications to relieve pain, and strategies to keep bones healthy.

Cannabis has known analgesic properties, and may be used to treat chronic pain from this condition. See Pain: chronic/severe/intractable for more information and references.

Additional Fibrous Dysplasia resources:
American Academy of Orthopaedic Surgeons: orthoinfo.aaos.org
Bone Tumor.org: www.bonetumor.org
Fibrous Dysplasia Foundation: www.fibrousdysplasia.org
Institute of Arthritis and Musculoskeletal and Skin Diseases: www.niams.nih.gov

Glaucoma

Glaucoma is a common disease of the eye that is usually caused by abnormally high fluid pressure, although it can also occur without increased pressure. Untreated, glaucoma can damage the optic nerve and lead to loss of vision and blindness. The National Eye Institute reports that African and Mexican Americans over age 40 and 60, respectively, as well as anyone with a family history of glaucoma, are at increased risk for glaucoma. There is no cure, and although there are medications and surgical procedures to treat glaucoma, any vision lost to the disease cannot be restored. Early studies in the 1970s and 80s showed that cannabis could reduce intraocular (within the eye) pressure and alleviate symptoms of glaucoma.[137, 263, 265–267, 541–546] The cannabinoid receptor CB1 is expressed at high levels in the human[538] and rat[539] eye, and topical application of a synthetic cannabinoid significantly decreased intraocular pressure in human glaucoma that resisted other treatments.[540] More recent research on cannabis and intraocular pressure confirms the earlier studies.[181, 537]

Additional Glaucoma resources:
American Glaucoma Society: www.americanglaucomasociety.net
American Optometric Association: www.aoa.org
BrightFocus Foundation: www.brightfocus.org
Glaucoma Research Foundation: www.glaucoma.org
National Eye Institute: www.nei.nih.gov
The Glaucoma Foundation: www.glaucomafoundation.org

Hepatitis C

Hepatitis C is an infection of the liver by the Hepatitis C virus (HCV) that causes inflammation and potentially cirrhosis or liver cancer. Symptoms also include joint pain, fatigue, nausea, anorexia, and depression. Hepatitis C can be transmitted to others through blood,[263, 267, 543, 546] commonly by needles, or congenitally, but it can also be sexually transmitted, or by sharing items that have come in contact with an infected person's blood. Severity of hepatitis C can range from mild, self-limited illness to chronic and serious lifelong illness that can be fatal. The US CDC estimates that 75-85% of people with HCV infection will develop a chronic illness; in 2009, approximately 3.2 million people in the United States had chronic HCV infections. Cannabinoids were effective at alleviating anorexia and nausea in Hepatitis C patients in two studies[489, 547] and helped patients to manage treatment-related side effects, which improved health and symptom outcomes.[547]

Additional Hepatitis C resources:
The American Liver Foundation: hepc.liverfoundation.org
Hepatitis Central: www.hepatitiscentral.com
HepC.com: www.hepc.com
US Centers for Disease Control and Prevention: www.cdc.gov
World Health Organization: www.who.int

Hospice/terminal illness

Individuals with terminal illness face special needs, and often opt for hospice care. According to Hospice of Southern Illinois, Inc. (www.hospice. org), hospice care focuses upon comfort and symptom management when a patient has a terminal illness with a prognosis of 6 months or less and when curative treatment is no longer possible or desired. The goal of hospice is to alleviate suffering and to support the patient emotionally, physically, and psychosocially to improve their quality of life. Cannabis is considered to be a safer pain and anxiety reducer than, for example, opioids,[551] and may provide symptom management for hospice and other terminally ill patients.

Additional Hospice resources:
American Hospice Foundation: americanhospice.org
Hospice: www.hospicenet.org
Hospice Directory: www.hospicedirectory.org
Hospice Foundation of America: hospicefoundation.org
International Association for Hospice & Palliative Care:
www.hospicecare.com
National Hospice and Palliative Care Organization: www.nhpco.org

Human Immunodeficiency Virus infection (see also AIDS)

The Human Immunodeficiency Virus (HIV) spreads throughout the immune system, predominantly affecting the T-helper (CD4) cells. Viruses are parasitic on their host cells (the host is the organism that the virus infects, in this case, the human) and rely upon them to reproduce themselves and infect other cells in the host's body, and then to be passed on to other hosts. HIV reproduces in the infected immune cells and kills them as it spreads to new cells—this destruction of immune cells makes the infected person more vulnerable to other types of infections, even from organisms that individuals with healthy immune systems can normally resist (known as "opportunistic" infections). HIV infection does progress over time, but it may reproduce in the body at very low levels for up to a decade, and if the patient is on antiretroviral therapy they may remain in this asymptomatic stage for multiple decades. Without treatment, most infected people will develop signs of HIV-related illness within 5-10 years. There is no known cure for HIV infection, and in many cases the amount of virus in the body eventually overwhelms the immune system to the point that opportunistic infections and cancers occur. This late stage of HIV infection is known as AIDS, the acquired immunodeficiency syndrome.

HIV is considered a sexually transmitted disease, but in fact is transmitted in several other ways as well: contaminated needles or syringes, contaminated medical equipment, or congenitally from an infected mother—generally, any manner in which certain infected body fluids (blood, penile, vaginal and rectal fluids, and breast milk) contact the mucous membranes or blood of a non-infected person. The US CDC estimates that at the end of 2011, approximately 1.2 million people in the United States were infected with HIV, about 14% of whom were unaware of the infection. HIV is a global epidemic – the World Health Organization and UNAIDS estimate that at the end of 2013, 35 million people in the world were living with HIV infections. During that year, about 2.1 million people became newly infected with the virus, and 1.5 million people died of AIDS-related causes. The number one related infection that kills HIV-infected people is tuberculosis.

In addition to the symptom relief afforded by cannabis (see AIDS), a research study also found that components of marijuana help decrease the amount of the virus, reduce inflammation, and slow progression of AIDS by modulating the host's immune system.[286] It is thought that HIV may spread in the host by causing inflammation of the gastrointestinal system that activates the immune system and allows for further infection of host cells. A study of immunodeficiency in macaque monkeys found that administration of THC protects the intestines from damage and inflammation, and potentially protects against further spread of the virus.[127] Azidothymidine (AZT) was the first antiretroviral drug created for HIV, but AIDS.gov reports that there have since been approximately 30 medications developed and approved to treat HIV/AIDS falling into five different classes. Each of the different classes of HIV drug affects the virus in a different way, so a patient will commonly take 3 different drugs from 2 different classes. Unfortunately, these medications can have debilitating side effects, including pain, diarrhea, and nausea. Cannabinoids have proven beneficial in easing side effects (see Treatment with AZT, chemotherapy, protease inhibitors, radiation therapy).

Additional Human Immunodeficiency Virus resources:

AIDS 2014: www.aids2014.org
AIDS.gov: www.aids.gov
AIDS.org: www.aids.org
AVERT: www.avert.org
UNAIDS: www.unaids.org
US Centers for Disease Control: www.cdc.gov
World Health Organization: www.who.int

Huntington's disease

According to the National Library of Medicine, Huntington's disease is a neurodegenerative disorder of the brain that is caused by mutations in the *HTT* gene. This means that children with a parent who has Huntington's disease have a 50/50 chance of inheriting the abnormality and developing the disease. Huntington's disease is characterized by uncontrolled, involuntary movements (known as chorea), emotional problems, and loss of cognition. People with Huntington's disease develop difficulties with every day activities such as walking, speaking, and swallowing, thinking and reasoning, and usually experience personality changes. Although the disease can begin at any age, it usually has onset in a person's thirties or forties, and life expectancy is approximately 15-20 years following disease onset. In the juvenile form of Huntington's disease, seizures occur in 30-50% of patients, and life expectancy is about 10-15 years following onset. The Huntington's Disease Society of America reports that about

20,000 people in the United States have Huntington's disease. There is no known cure and treatment comprises administration of medications to relieve symptoms.

Cannabis has neuroprotective effects that may prove beneficial in treating Huntington's disease (see Tables 1 and 2). In a rat model, the cannabis-based medicine Sativex had neuroprotective effects capable of delaying Huntington's disease.[88, 555] Meisel and Friedman[554] found that cannabis alleviated anxiety and depression, improved sleep, and in one subject, slightly improved motor skills.

Additional Huntington's disease resources:
Alzheimer's Association: www.alz.org
Huntington's Disease Association England and Wales: hda.org.uk
Family Caregiver Alliance: caregiver.org
Huntington's Disease Society of America: www.hdsa.org
National Institutes of Neurological Disorders and Stroke:
www.ninds.nih.gov
The International Huntington Association: www.huntington-assoc.com

Hydrocephalus

Hydrocephalus is a condition in which excess fluid accumulates in the brain, potentially causing harmful pressure on brain tissues. Hydrocephalus can be present at birth (congenital) and caused by genetic abnormalities or by circumstances that occur during fetal development. Acquired hydrocephalus develops at birth or at any age afterward, and can be caused by injury or disease. The National Institute of Neurological Disorders and Stroke indicates that about 1-2 infants out every 1000 are born with hydrocephalus. Symptoms of hydrocephalus depend on age and disease progression. Infants typically have an unusually large head size, and may have vomiting, sleepiness, irritability, downward deviation of the eyes, and seizures. The skulls of children and adults cannot expand for the extra fluid, and symptoms may include headache, vomiting, nausea, vision disturbances, downward deviation of eyes, poor balance and coordination, problems walking, urinary incontinence, lethargy, irritability, memory loss, and personality or cognition changes. Hydrocephalus is usually treated by surgery to install a shunt.

Cannabis has analgesic, anti-nausea, anti-emetic, and anti-seizure properties that may make it useful in the treatment of symptoms of hydrocephalus. See Tables 1 and 2 as well as the sections on Migraine; Nausea; Seizures; Vomiting: intractable for more information and references.

Additional Hydrocephalus resources:
Hydrocephalus association: www.hydroassoc.org
National Institute of Neurological Disorders and Stroke:
www.ninds.nih.gov

Inflammatory bowel disease
(IBD—see also Crohn's disease)

Inflammatory bowel disease comprises several conditions that are characterized by chronic or recurring inflammation of the gastrointestinal tract. Chronic inflammation arises because the immune system reacts to food and intestinal flora (normal bacteria) as foreign substances; immune complexes attack the cells of the intestine and can cause severe symptoms that progress over time. The US CDC reports that the two most common IBDs are ulcerative colitis, in which only the large intestine is affected, and Crohn's disease, in which the entire digestive tract is affected. Both Crohn's disease and ulcerative colitis are serious conditions accompanied by debilitating symptoms including diarrhea, anorexia and weight loss, fatigue, and bleeding that may lead to anemia. Surgery is required in a large number of cases.

Cannabis is known for anti-inflammatory properties, and in mouse[111] and rat[56] models of IBD cannabinoids reduced colitis. A study of cannabidiol derivatives on a mouse model showed that intestinal motility (intestinal contractions that propel fecal matter) was inhibited by acting on the peripheral nervous system[23], and the authors suggest that complex disorders such as inflammatory bowel disease and cystic fibrosis may benefit from development of cannabis-based medicines. IBD patients who are treated with cannabis report improvement in general health, social functioning and ability to work, and reduction of pain and depression.[559] A survey of 313 IBD patients who used cannabis to alleviate symptoms[238] found that abdominal pain and cramping were reduced in 83.9% and 76.8%, respectively, joint pain was relieved in 48.2%, and diarrhea was relieved in 28.6%, however, use of cannabis for more than 6 months was also associated with higher risk of surgery in Crohn's disease patients; this study is consistent with that of Lal and colleagues.[523] A survey of 292 IBD patients[558] found similar results, indicating that cannabis reduced abdominal pain, appetite loss, nausea and diarrhea.

Additional Inflammatory bowel disease resources:
American Gastroenterological Association: www.gastro.org
Crohn's & Colitis: www.crohnsandcolitisinfo.com
Crohn's & Colitis Foundation of America: www.cfa.org
Crohn's & Me: www.crohnsandme.com
National Institute of Diabetes and Digestive and Kidney Diseases: www.niddk.nih.gov
US Centers for Disease Control and Prevention: www.cdc.gov

Interstitial cystitis

Interstitial cystitis is also known as painful bladder syndrome. The National Kidney and Urologic Diseases Information Clearinghouse indicates that the symptoms and severity of this condition vary so much by individual that it is thought to be more than one disease. The condition is characterized by discomfort, pressure, tenderness, or intense pain in the bladder and pelvic area, and can be accompanied by an urgent and/or frequent need to urinate. The pain intensity can change as the bladder fills and empties, and for women, the symptoms may increase during menstruation, and vaginal intercourse may be painful. Interstitial cystitis/painful bladder syndrome is not caused by an infection or urinary stones, although the symptoms may mimic bacterial infection. The cause of the condition is unknown, but often co-occurs with irritable bowel syndrome and fibromyalgia, and is thought to be part of a more general inflammatory condition throughout the body. Treatments are focused on symptom relief and include measures such as bladder distention, bladder instillation (filling and emptying the bladder with a medication solution), electrical nerve stimulation of the bladder, dietary alteration and cessation of tobacco smoking, and several oral medications including those to relieve pain. In cases with disabling pain and when all other treatments fail, surgery may be an option.

Cannabis has anti-inflammatory and analgesic properties that may help to reduce inflammation and, particularly, pain symptoms of interstitial cystitis. See Tables 1 and 2 and the section on Pain: chronic/severe/intractable for more information and references.

Additional Interstitial cystitis references:
American Urological Association:
www.auanet.org
IC Network: www.ic-network.com
The National Kidney Foundation:
www.kidney.org
The National Kidney and Urologic Diseases Information Clearinghouse: kidney. niddk.nih.gov

Migraine

Migraine is a headache disorder, and the World Health Organization estimates that some 47% of adults age 18-65 years worldwide may suffer from a headache disorder. Headache disorders include migraine, tension-type headaches, cluster headaches, and medication overuse headaches. The Migraine Research Foundation describes migraine as a neurological syndrome, characterized by a suite of symptoms including severe, recurring, intense throbbing pain of one or both sides of the head. A migraine may last up to 72 hours, and may have additional symptoms such as vision disturbance, dizziness, nausea and vomiting, tingling or numbness of face or extremities, and extreme sensitivity to light, sound, touch, and smell. The symptoms can be sufficiently severe that patients visit the emergency room; additionally, side effects or reactions from migraine medications can also send a patient to the ER. Both children and adults can suffer from migraine. The Migraine Research Foundation estimates that approximately 36 million people in the United

States suffer from migraine. Headache disorders are a considerable cost to society. Work and school days can be lost because of severe headaches. Treatment for migraine includes medications for symptom relief and also to reduce number of attacks, as well as non-drug therapies such as biofeedback, relaxation, acupuncture, exercise, and lifestyle changes focused upon proper sleep and diet habits.

Reports from patients with migraine indicate that cannabis can help to relieve migraine pain and other symptoms.[478, 563, 566, 567] Cannabis activates CB1 receptors in the brain and may help to correct endogenous cannabinoid deficiencies that contribute to migraine.[197] In a rat model, THC helped to suppress cortical spreading depression, a phenomenon that may cause or contribute to migraine.[560]

Additional Migraine resources:
American Migraine Foundation: www.americanmigrainefoundation.org
Migraine Research Foundation: migraineresearchfoundation.org
National Institute of Neurological Disorders and Stroke:
www.ninds.nih.gov
National Migraine Association: www.migraines.org
World Health Organization: www.who.int

Multiple sclerosis

Multiple sclerosis (MS) is a debilitating and disabling degenerative disease of the central nervous system. MS is thought to result from an abnormal process in which the person's own immune cells attack and destroy the myelin sheath that covers and protects nerves. Scar tissue forms over the nerve and the signals that travel to and from the brain and spinal cord are disrupted. The National Multiple Sclerosis Society indicates that the exact target of this immune attack is unknown, so experts currently consider the disease to be "immune-mediated" rather than "autoimmune".

The National Multiple Sclerosis Society describes four different courses of MS, each of which has its own characteristic symptoms and ranges in severity. All four courses of MS involve myelin and nerve damage, brain lesions, and spinal cord lesions. Symptoms of MS vary between and within the four courses, but the most common are fatigue and weakness, tingling and numbness, spasticity, pain, difficulty walking, vision problems, bladder and bowel dysfunction, sexual problems, reduced cognitive functions, and depression and irritability. Other symptoms may include speech and swallowing difficulties, seizures or tremors, respiration problems, itching or burning sensations, headache, and hearing loss.

- *Relapsing-remitting MS* (RRMS) is the most common form of the disease (85% of cases), and is characterize by flare-ups of inflammatory attacks on the myelin sheaths and on the nerves themselves. The flare-ups are followed by periods of remission that have partial or complete improvement of symptoms until the next flare-up. The disease can occur at any age, but is usually diagnosed in young people between 20 and 40 years of age, and is two to three times more common in women than men. People with RRMS usually end up transitioning into secondary-progressive MS after 10 or more years.

- *Secondary-progressive MS* (SPMS) follows from RRMS, and thus is the second most common form of MS. SPMS has fewer of the inflammation attacks seen in RRMS, and more progressive nerve damage or loss. Patients may or may not continue to have remission periods.

- *Primary-progressive MS* (PPMS) is characterized more by nerve degeneration rather than inflammation. Patients have fewer brain lesions and more spinal cord lesions than in RRMS, and there are fewer inflammatory cells. The disease is progressive, meaning that symptoms gradually get worse, and there are no remission periods. Average age of onset is between 40 and 60 years of age, and both sexes are equally likely to develop the disease. Mobility problems are common in PPMS, patients often require assistance with daily activities, and ability to work outside the home can be limited.

- The least common form of MS is progressive-relapsing MS (PRMS), which occurs in approximately 5% of patients. PRMS is progressive like PPMS, but there may be occasional relapses similar to that in RRMS.

Treatments for MS involve reduction of disease activity and disease progression, as well as management of symptoms and rehabilitation therapies. Twelve medications have been approved by the US Food and Drug Administration for disease modification, but these function to reduce inflammation and thus are only truly effective for RRMS, SPMS, and PRMS. The National Multiple Sclerosis Society reports that there are currently no approved medications for disease modification of PPMS.

Many of the scientific studies referred to in this report focus on patients' perceived ability of cannabis to reduce symptoms.[491, 579, 580, 582, 583, 585, 591] Research on animals and humans increasingly shows that herbal cannabinoids help reduce spasticity, tremor, and other motor symptoms of MS,[171, 184, 216, 276, 278, 279, 281–283, 568, 573, 577, 578, 584, 588] as well as pain,[77, 225, 235, 236, 574] bladder dysfunction, [210, 575, 581, 592] and vision,[587, 589] and cognition[476] problems. Several studies have found that cannabis can modulate the inflammatory processes that are so harmful in MS[59, 71, 293, 586], and inhibit neurodegeneration.[22, 299] A 3 year clinical trial found that oral THC was able to significantly slow neurodegeneration in individuals who had non-progressive forms of MS.[298]

> Additional Multiple Sclerosis resources:
> MultipleSclerosis.com: www.multiplesclerosis.com
> National Institute of Neurological Disorders and Stroke:
> www.ninds.nih.gov
> National Multiple Sclerosis Society www.nationalmssociety.org
> The Multiple Sclerosis Association of America: www.mymsaa.org

Muscle spasms (see Spasticity/spinal cord damage)
Muscular dystrophy

Muscular dystrophies comprise a group of diseases characterized by progressive muscle weakness that leads to decreased mobility and reduced quality of life. The US CDC describes 8 major types of muscular dystrophy, but there are many more, each involving different muscle groups and other body parts. Muscles in any part of the body can be affected, and depending upon the type of muscular dystrophy, other organ systems may be involved. Secondary damage to bones due to muscular inactivity and to medications may occur. Mental and emotional health may also suffer because of the disease, because of medications used to treat the disease, or due to the stresses of living with the disease. All of the muscular dystrophies are reported by CDC to be relatively rare (from about

15 cases per 100,000 US males in 2007 for Duchenne/Becker muscular dystrophy to fewer than 1 case per 100,000 people in Northern England for Emery-Dreifuss muscular dystrophy), and all are caused by deleterious genetic variants.

There is currently no known cure for any of the muscular dystrophies. Treatment regimens for muscular dystrophies depend upon the type of disease and its manifestation in an individual. As a progressive disease, muscular dystrophy is characterized by stages from pre-symptomatic, in which an individual is showing no signs yet, all the way to late non-ambulatory, in which mobility is significantly limited, and other organ systems are likely impaired. Steroid medications are used to help slow muscle damage and maintain strength for as long as possible, and other medications may be required to treat bone, heart, and digestive issues. Opiates may be prescribed for the chronic pain that accompanies lack of mobility and muscle spasms. Rehabilitation therapies and assistive devices such as wheelchairs can aid mobility.

With its analgesic, anti-spasmodic, and anti-anxiety properties, cannabis can benefit muscular dystrophy patients (see Tables 1 and 2 and the sections on Pain; Spasticity; see also Chapter 4, Anxiety). Because the respiratory system may be compromised in several types of muscular dystrophy, smoking is contra-indicated, but vaporization and ingestion of cannabis or essential oils are other acceptable methods of administration.

Additional Muscular Dystrophy resources:
American Academy of Orthopaedic Surgeons: orthoinfo.aaos.org
FSH Society: www.fshsociety.org
Muscular Dystrophy Association: www.mda.org
Muscular Dystrophy Campaign: www.muscular-dystrophy.org
Myotonic Dystrophy Foundation: www.myotonic.org
Parent Project Muscular Dystrophy: www.parentprojectmd.org
US Centers for Disease Control and Prevention: www.cdc.gov

Myasthenia gravis

Myasthenia gravis is a neuromuscular disease characterized by weakness of the voluntary muscles. Weakness increases when the muscle is active, and improves after rest. The muscles that control eye movement, eyelids, facial expressions, chewing, talking, and swallowing are typically involved, and muscles that control breathing and movement of neck and limbs may also be affected. The National Institute of Neurological Disorders and Stroke indicates that the disease is a chronic autoimmune disorder caused by a defect in the transmission of nerve impulses to muscles. The immune system produces antibodies, which are normally supposed to fight against foreign invaders that mistakenly attack and block, alter, or even destroy some of the nerve receptors. The thymus gland, which is important in the development of the immune system, has been found to be enlarged and abnormal in adults who have myasthenia gravis, although the exact role of the thymus gland in myasthenia gravis is not yet understood.

Myasthenia gravis can occur at any age, but it most commonly affects women under 40 and men over 60. Symptoms of myasthenia gravis vary in type and severity, and include weakness of eye muscles, difficulty swallowing and speaking, drooping of eyelids, double vision, unstable gait, change in facial expression, and weakness of arms, hands, fingers, legs, and neck. In individuals with affected respiratory muscles, there can be "myasthenic crises", in which the breathing muscles weaken to the point that a respiratory is required for ventilation. There is of yet no cure for myasthenia gravis, but treatment includes medications to improve neuromuscular transmission, to increase muscle strength, and to suppress the immune system. There can be major side effects of some of these medications. Surgical removal of the thyroid is sometimes effective, as is a procedure in which part of the blood that has the antibodies is removed and replaced.

Cannabis has anti-inflammatory, neuroprotective, and anti-anxiety properties, and may be useful to treat both the autoimmune and neurodegenerative issues of the disease as well as associated anxiety and pain. Because the respiratory system is involved, smoking of cannabis is contraindicated, but oral and vaporized cannabis is an acceptable method of administration. See Tables 1 and 2 and sections on Pain: chronic/severe/intractable; Peripheral neuropathy and in Chapter 4 Anxiety disorders; Autoimmune disorders for more information and references.

Additional Myasthenia gravis resources:
Muscular Dystrophy Association: mda.org
Myasthenia Gravis Association: www.myaware.org
Myasthenia Gravis Foundation of America: www.myasthenia.org
The National Institute of Neurological Disorders and Stroke:
www.ninds.nih.gov

Myoclonus

Myoclonus is the sudden, involuntary jerking of a muscle or group of muscles. Myoclonic jerks can be positive (caused by muscle contraction) or negative (caused by muscle relaxation). Myoclonic jerks may occur singly or multiply, with or without a pattern, and are unable to be controlled. The National Institute of Neurological Disorders and Stroke describes the simplest forms of myoclonus as being like a hiccup or the twitches experienced while following asleep: a muscle twitch followed by relaxation. More severe cases of myoclonus can distort movement and limit eating, talking, and/or walking. Myoclonus that occurs during sleep can affect the person's ability to get sufficient rest. The National Institute of Neurological Disorders and Stroke details the 8 main types of myoclonus, although there are many more. These are beyond the scope of this report and are not described here; interested readers are referred to www.ninds.nih.gov for more information.

Myoclonus has a wide range of potential causes: infections, injuries, strokes, brain tumors, kidney or liver failure, lipid storage diseases, poisons, oxygen deprivation, and in combination with other neurological disorders such as epilepsy, multiple sclerosis, Parkinson's disease, Alzheimer's disease, or Creutzfeldt-Jacob disease. Other than in cases of injury to the brain and spinal cord, myoclonus is a central nervous system disturbance, with several brain regions involved. It is thought that abnormalities in receptors for neurotransmitters (the chemicals that transmit signals in the brain and throughout the nervous system) may contribute to some forms of myoclonus. Treatment of myoclonus focuses on symptom reduction, typically with anti-seizure drugs. Tolerance may be developed over time to some of these drugs, and some may have adverse side effects.

Cannabis has antispasmodic, anti-seizure, and sedative properties that may be beneficial in treating myoclonus. See Tables 1 and 2 and sections on Muscle spasms; Seizures and Chapter 4 Sleep disturbances for further information and references.

Additional Myoclonus resources:
American Sleep Association: www.sleepassociation.org
Epilepsy Foundation: www.epilepsy.com
National Institute of Neurological Disorders and Stroke: www.ninds.nih.gov
The Movement Disorder Society: www.movementdisorders.org

Nail-patella syndrome

Nail-patella is a rare genetic disorder that can be inherited from an affected parent, or that may occur from a new mutation in the associated gene. It is also frequently known as Fong's disease. Although it is unknown exactly how the genetic defects lead to the syndrome, according to the National Library of Medicine early embryonic development of limbs, kidneys, and eyes is affected. People with nail-patella syndrome almost always have absent or underdeveloped and disfigured nails and patellae (kneecaps). Other parts of the skeleton are also commonly affected, with elbows, knees, and pelvic bones abnormally shaped, sometimes causing mobility problems and pain. Kidney disease is possible, and may progress to kidney failure, and increased pressure of the eyes (glaucoma) can lead to blindness. Approximately 1 in 50,000 individuals is thought to have nail-patella syndrome. Cannabis compound THC has been shown to reduce pressure in the eye, and cannabinoids have significant anti-inflammatory and pain relief properties for arthritis and kidney inflammation. See Tables 1 and 2 and sections on Arthritis; Chronic renal failure; Glaucoma; Pain/chronic/severe/intractable).

Additional Nail-patella syndrome resources:
Nail Patella Syndrome Worldwide: www.npsw.org
National Organization for Rare Diseases: www.rarediseases.org

Nausea

Nausea is a common response to conditions such as pregnancy, motion sickness, and extreme emotions such as fear and anxiety, but it can also be a symptom of many debilitating diseases, as well as a significant side effect of certain medications and radiation therapy. Sharkey and colleagues[662] provide an excellent and current (although technical) discussion of the present state of knowledge of the effects of cannabis, via the cannabinoid receptors and endocannabinoid system, on nausea and vomiting. To very briefly summarize, CB1 receptors are located in regions of the brain that are involved in regulating nausea and vomiting. Substances that stimulate CB1 receptors can evoke nausea and vomiting in humans and in animals that are capable of vomiting. Endocannabinoids are thought to be capable of acting at the CB1 receptor to limit its activation, and thus to suppress the nausea and vomiting impulses. Cannabinoids, particularly THC, appear to act in a similar manner to the endocannabinoids to suppress nausea and vomiting in humans.[120, 128, 140, 168, 177, 179, 600, 663, 664] In animal models, cannabinoids were effective inhibitors of induced nausea responses.[85, 86, 102, 103, 169, 258] A paradoxical effect of cannabis, however, has been noted following heavy chronic cannabis use, especially in young people. Known as "cannabinoid hyperemesis syndrome", individuals experience abdominal pain, recurrent nausea, and intractable cyclic vomiting that may be relieved by hot baths and showers.[358, 363] Sharkey and colleagues[662] indicate that the syndrome appears to be a relatively recent phenomenon, potentially due to either buildup of some toxin derived from the cannabis (perhaps due to new horticultural practices) or from downregulation of the CB1 receptors following high exposure.

Neurofibromatosis

Neurofibromatosis comprises three different genetic disorders that are characterized by tumor formation in the nervous system. The National Institute of Neurological Disorders and Stroke indicates that the disorders are classified into three types: neurofibromatosis type 1 (NF1, also known as von Recklinghausen's disease), neurofibromatosis type 2 (NF2), and schwannomatosis. Neurofibromatosis can occur in anyone, and is thought to affect about 100,000 Americans. The most common type is

NF1. Children with NF1 have larger than normal head circumference and shorter than normal stature. Hydrocephalus (buildup of fluid in the brain) may occur, and headache and epilepsy are common. There can be congenital heart defects, high blood pressure, and constricted, blocked, or damaged blood vessels. Poor learning and academic skills are common, as is attention deficit hyperactivity disorder. Up to 5 percent of the tumors may become cancerous in NF1. There is no known way to prevent growth of neurofibroma tumors, and surgery may be possible in only some cases. If the tumors become malignant, anti-cancer treatments may be required.

NF2 is reported as rare, affecting about 1 in 25,000 people. The condition is characterized by slow-growing tumors (schwannomas) on the eighth cranial nerve, which typically disturb hearing and balance.

There may be other schwannomas in nerves throughout the body. The tumors grow and can cause damage to other nerves and the brain stem, which in turn may cause serious disability. People with NF2 are at increased risk for developing other types of nervous system tumors, and they may also develop cataracts or retinal changes that affect vision. Tumors can also cause peripheral neuropathy and associated numbness and weakness of extremities. Treatment depends on tumor size and location and other symptoms. Surgery may be required when possible.

Schwannomatosis is also rare and is similar to NF2 except that there is no eighth cranial nerve involvement, and multiple schwannomas occur throughout the body. Schwannomatosis is very painful, and compression of nerves may lead to peripheral neuropathy. The treatment is surgical management of tumors when possible, and management of pain when not possible.

Cannabis has anti-tumor, anti-inflammatory, anti-seizure, and analgesic properties to make it beneficial for the treatment of tumor formation, inflammation, seizures and headaches associated with neurofibromatosis. See Tables 1 and 2 and sections on Cancer; Migraine; Pain: chronic/severe/intractable; Peripheral neuropathy; Seizures for more information and references.

Additional Neurofibromatosis resources:
National Institute of Neurological Disorders and Stroke:
www.ninds.nih.gov

Pain: chronic/severe/intractable

Chronic pain is a condition in which nerves signal pain for extensive periods of time, from weeks to years, even in the absence of an immediate injury. A common theme with most of the debilitating conditions discussed in this manual is the presence of chronic pain, often intractable to conventional medical treatments. Additionally, pain as a side effect of chemotherapy can be so significant that patients sometimes opt to discontinue their therapy regimen. The National Institute of Neurological Disorders and Stroke indicates that treatments for chronic pain include medications, local electrical stimulation, brain stimulation and surgery as well as nontraditional therapies such as acupuncture, psychotherapy, relaxation, biofeedback, and behavior modification. Cannabinoids are also receiving increased scientific attention as effective analgesics.

Surveys of patients suffering chronic pain conditions indicate that cannabis can have powerful perceived analgesic effects.[239, 603, 606, 611, 615, 618, 620, 665] Research on both acute and chronic pain indicates that cannabinoids operate on the endocannabinoid system to modulate pain in the same manner in which opioids act, and may be co-administered with opioids to reduce the necessary dose of opioid required for the same effect.[204, 228] Laboratory studies in animal models show that cannabinoids act upon the CB2 receptors[609] and/or on the glycine receptors of the spine[98] to modulate chronic pain. In vitro research also showed that the glycine receptors are activated by cannabinoids.[25, 614] Chemotherapy-induced pain in laboratory rats was alleviated by treatment with cannabidiol.[95] In human subjects, smoked marijuana has been found to increase pain tolerance,[230] and a large number of clinical trials have found that cannabinoids are effective analgesics in chronic pain conditions.[40, 96, 147, 154, 206, 207, 215, 218, 221, 222, 224, 226, 231, 236, 237, 240–242, 604, 607, 608, 610, 612, 616, 617, 619]

Additional Pain resources:
American Chronic Pain Association: theacpa.org
National Fibromyalgia & Chronic Pain Association: www.fmpcaware.org
National Institute of Neurological Disorders and Stroke:
www.ninds.nih.gov

Pancreatitis

The National Library of Medicine describes pancreatitis as an inflammation of the pancreas that can be acute (of sudden onset and short duration) or chronic (progressive development and extended duration). Both forms are serious and can lead to complications, although acute pancreatitis can improve or heal in a few days with intravenous fluid, antibiotic, and analgesic treatments. A common cause of acute pancreatitis is gallstones. Chronic pancreatitis leads to permanent damage, and can be caused by excessive alcohol consumption, inherited disorders such as cystic fibrosis, autoimmune disorders, high blood levels of calcium or fats, and medications such as those prescribed for HIV/AIDS patients. Treatment for chronic pancreatitis also relies on IV fluids and analgesic medications, in addition to dietary and lifestyle modifications. Symptoms of both types of pancreatitis include pain, nausea, and vomiting, and chronic pancreatitis leads to weight loss and potentially to wasting. Cannabis may benefit patients with pancreatitis through its anti-inflammatory, anti-nausea and anti-emetic, analgesic, and appetite stimulating properties. In HIV/AIDS patients on three different types of antiretroviral therapy (azidothymidine, azidothymidine/dideoxycytidine, or dideoxyinosine), clinical indicators of pancreatitis improved in the dideocyinosine group who used either Marinol (a synthetic version of THC) or herbal cannabis.[622]

Additional Pancreatitis resources:
American Gastroenterological Association: www.gastro.org
The Pancreas Center: pancreasmd.org

Parkinson's disease

Parkinson's disease is a neurological disease of the brain that is slowly progressive, and is characterized by an inability to regulate movement and emotions. Parkinson's disease occurs when the brain stops producing dopamine, a chemical that relays messages in the brain to help control movements. The National Parkinson Foundation indicates that after 60-80% of the cells that produce dopamine are damaged, the brain can no longer regulate body movement and motor symptoms begin to appear. These symptoms include tremor, shaking, or twitching of limbs, stiffness that does not go away with movement, difficulty moving or walking, change in voice or facial expression (called "masking"), dizziness or fainting, difficulty standing up straight, sudden movements during sleep, loss of sense of smell, and constipation not attributed to dietary or medicine factors. There is currently no cure for Parkinson's disease. Treatments include medications to help replenish dopamine or to take the place of dopamine, surgeries in some cases, and rehabilitation therapies. The anti-inflammatory and antioxidant properties of cannabinoids are thought to help reduce neurodegeneration. In animal models, THC and CBC helped to delay progression of neurodegeneration[61, 191] and THC reduced motor symptoms.[191] An anonymous survey of Parkinson's patients indicated that 25% used cannabis because of its perceived benefits.[623] Studies on human patients with Parkinson's disease indicate that smoked cannabis can significantly improve motor symptoms, pain, and sleep.[227] Cannabidiol has been found to reduce REM sleep behavior disorder,[33] and to provide higher well-being and quality of life to patients.[35]

Additional Parkinson's disease resources:
American Parkinson Disease Association: www.adpaparkinson.org
Bachmann-Strauss Dystonia & Parkinson Foundation, Inc.:
www.dystonia-parkinsons.org
National Institute of Neurological Disorders and Stroke:
www.ninds.nih.gov
National Parkinson Foundation: www.parkinson.org
NIH Senior Health: nihseniorhealth.gov
Parkinson's Disease Foundation: www.pdf.org
Parkinsons.org: www.parkinsons.org

Peripheral neuropathy

Peripheral neuropathy results from damage to one or more peripheral nerves (those outside of the brain and spinal cord). The US National Institute of Neurological Disorders and Stroke (NINDS) estimates that some 20 million people in the US have some form of peripheral neuropathy. The causes of peripheral neuropathy are many and varied: most common is trauma from injury or repetitive stress, but diseases, exposure to medications, toxins, or heavy alcohol consumption are also frequent causes. Less frequent forms of peripheral neuropathy may be inherited or from new genetic mutations. Many of the debilitating conditions for which marijuana is authorized can cause peripheral neuropathy: diabetes, autoimmune diseases, kidney disease, cancers, and infections such as HIV can all cause peripheral neuropathy. Additionally, medications used to treat cancers, AIDS/HIV, epilepsy and even cardiovascular conditions can cause peripheral neuropathy as a side effect.

The peripheral nervous system is responsible for communicating with the central nervous system (brain and spinal cord). Signaling between the peripheral and central nervous systems is key to the ability to move (motor nerves), to utilize the senses (sensory nerves), and for function of our organ systems (autonomic nerves). The NINDS indicates that over 100 types of peripheral neuropathy have been described. These neuropathies may affect only one type of nerves, or may affect all three. Additionally, the neuropathy may be limited to a relatively small portion of the body, or may be systemic. Symptoms of peripheral neuropathy can be transient, such as those caused by medication side effects that resolve when the medication is discontinued, but can also be long-lasting or permanent, such as those arising from genetic conditions or from leprosy.

Symptoms of peripheral neuropathy can be relatively mild, such as numbness, tingling, prickling sensations, or muscle weakness. A distorted sense of touch can lead to extreme sensitivity and pain in response to normally non-painful stimuli. Damage to the sensory nerves can also lead to an inability to feel sensations and to know if an injury is occurring. Symptoms can also be severe, and include burning pain, muscle wasting, cramps and muscle twitching, decreased reflexes, paralysis, and even respiratory difficulties or organ failures. Peripheral neuropathies that affect the autonomic nervous system can impair digestion, urination, and heart and gland functions.

Treatments for peripheral neuropathies depend upon the cause and type of neuropathy. For damage caused by medications, toxins, or infections, it may be possible to eliminate or reduce the underlying cause, and allow nerves to regenerate. Lifestyle changes to manage weight, exercise, and avoiding toxic substances and alcohol and tobacco can also be helpful. Dietary management is important for people with diabetic neuropathy. For neuropathies caused by inflammatory and autoimmune systems, there are medications to help control inflammation and immune activity. There are also several types of treatments aimed at symptom management, particularly pain. Drug therapy can range from over-the-counter pain medications to opioids for intractable pain. Surgery may be helpful for neuropathies such as carpal tunnel syndrome. The NINDS also describes a non-invasive therapy called transcutaneous electrical nerve stimulation (TENS), in which electrodes are attached to the skin and electrical current is passed through to help relieve pain – this is described to be particularly helpful with diabetic peripheral neuropathy.

In addition to studies cited for the various debilitating conditions that may cause peripheral neuropathy, research has focused specifically on the ability of cannabinoids for neuroprotection and to ease neuropathic pain. In rats, CBD was able to protect motor and sensory neurons, and to preserve signaling[80] and to reduce pain and nerve damage associated with diabetes.[212] Other studies on rat models indicated that cannabinoids were beneficial in relieving pain.[40, 213] Cannabis was also shown to have neuroprotective effects and to help with nerve regeneration in a recent human study.[608] Several human studies have found cannabinoids to reduce neuropathic pain,[241, 242, 626] including that caused by HIV,[205, 218, 233] multiple sclerosis,[225] and trauma.[207] A systematic review of effectiveness of cannabis extracts for management of chronic nonmalignant neuropathic pain found that cannabinoids may be effective at relieving pain when other methods fail.[209]

Additional Peripheral neuropathy resources:
American Diabetes Association: www.diabetes.org
American Podiatric Medical Association: www.apma.org
Cancer.net: www.cancer.net
National Foundation for Celiac Awareness: www.celiaccentral.org
National Institute of Neurological Disorders and Stroke:
www.ninds.nih.gov
The Foundation for Peripheral Neuropathy: www.foundationforpn.org
The Neuropathy Association: www.neuropathy.org
The Neuropathy Support Network: www.neuropathysupportnetwork.org

Post-traumatic stress disorder (PTSD)

Post-traumatic stress disorder, or PTSD, is an anxiety disorder that develops after someone experiences a situation in which physical harm or the threat of physical harm occurred. The National Institute of Mental Health (NIMH) describes PTSD as a changed or damaged "fight-or-flight" response that helps us to defend against or avoid danger: individuals with PTSD may have stress or fright emotions evoked even when no danger is present. PTSD symptoms do not go away within a short time after the traumatic event is over, but instead last more than a few weeks and become an ongoing problem that affects the person's ability to function in regular life. Although current research is underway to elucidate the mechanisms of brain function and genetics that can lead to PTSD, environmental, personality, and cognitive factors are also thought to be instrumental in causing PTSD. PTSD can occur at any age, and women are reported to be more likely to suffer the disorder.

The NIMH groups PTSD symptoms into three categories:

- *Re-experiencing* symptoms include nightmares, frightening thoughts, and flashbacks, in which the trauma is relived repeatedly. Flashbacks can cause physical reactions such as sweating and heart racing.

- *Avoidance* symptoms include staying away from anything that reminds the person of the traumatic event, feelings of emotional numbness, guilt, depression, or worry, difficulties remembering the traumatic event, and loss of interest in formerly pleasurable activities.

- *Hyperarousal* symptoms include feeling tense or edgy, being easily startled, having angry outbursts, and difficulty sleeping.

PTSD is usually treated by psychotherapy and/or medications. Psychotherapy helps people to understand their symptoms and to learn new ways to react to events that trigger the symptoms. Medications help to control depression and feelings of anxiety, anger and numbness, but they can have side effects. Surveys of PTSD patients indicate that cannabis can also relieve symptoms of depression, anxiety, anger, and numbness.[628, 629] Two studies found THC[627] and CBD[30] to be useful in PTSD symptom reduction. A case study and review of PTSD patients indicates that cannabinoids may help to reduce panic and flashbacks[288] via interaction with the endocannabinoid system.

Additional Post-traumatic stress disorder resources:
American Psychiatric Association:
www.psychiatry.org
American Psychological Association: www.apa.org
Anxiety Disorders Association of America: www.adaa.org
Gateway to Post Traumatic Stress Disorder Information:
www.ptsdinfo.org
National Alliance for the Mentally Ill: www.nami.org
National Institute of Mental Health: www.nimh.nih.gov
US Department of Veterans Affairs: www.ptsd.va.gov

Seizures (see Epilepsy)

Sjögren's syndrome

Sjögren's syndrome is an autoimmune disorder characterized by inflammatory response in which immune cells attack the moisture-producing cells of the body, especially in the tear and saliva glands. Symptoms vary in intensity, but patients have irritation and gritty or burning sensations in the eyes along with a dry mouth and swelling of glands around neck and face. Nasal passages, throat, vagina, and skin may also be dry. The American College of Rheumatology indicates that potentially up to 3.1 million adults may have Sjögren's syndrome. Persons of any age can be affected, but usually the symptoms appear between ages 45 and 55, and 10 times as many women as men are affected.

There are two types of Sjögren's syndrome. Primary Sjögren's syndrome occurs in people that have no other autoimmune disorder, while secondary Sjögren's syndrome occurs in people who have a disease such as systemic lupus erythematosus or rheumatoid arthritis. About half of Sjögren's syndrome patients have rheumatoid arthritis or lupus. The decreased tears and saliva cause patients to be at risk for eye and mouth infections, damage to the cornea, increased dental decay, and gingivitis.

There can also be episodes of painful swelling in the saliva glands. In patients with either primary or secondary Sjögren's syndrome, pain, stiffness, and swelling of joint areas may occur, along with arm and leg rashes, and inflammation of lungs, liver, and kidney. Numbness, tingling, and weakness may also be present.

Sjögren's syndrome is treated by addressing the symptoms. Artificial tears, medications, and regular dental care are all common treatments. Corticosteroids or immunosuppressive medications may be necessary in some cases.

Cannabis has anti-inflammatory and immunomodulatory properties that have been shown to be helpful against autoimmune disorders. Additionally, the analgesic properties of cannabis can help to relieve joint and muscle pain. See Tables 1 and 2 and the sections on Arthritis, Pain: chronic/severe/intractable, and Chapter 4 Autoimmune disorders for more information and references.

Additional Sjögren's syndrome resources:
American College of Rheumatology: www.rheumatology.org
Arthritis Foundation: www.arthritis.org
National Library of Medicine: www.nlm.nih.gov
Sjögren's Syndrome Foundation: www.sjogrens.org

Spasticity/spinal cord damage

Spasticity can result from damage to nerves caused by disease processes (see Amyotrophic Lateral Sclerosis; Huntington's Disease; Multiple Sclerosis) or from trauma to nerves or spinal cord (see also Peripheral Neuropathy). Research on animals and humans increasingly shows that herbal cannabinoids help reduce spasticity and tremors associated with various conditions.[171, 184, 216, 276, 278-283, 568, 573, 577, 578, 588, 594] Spinal cord injuries are also associated with musculoskeletal pain and chronic, neuropathic pain that may be difficult to treat.[211, 595] Damage to the spinal cord can permanently alter sensory perception, motor ability and organ function in areas of the body below the level of the injury. These changes can drastically affect lifestyle and perceived quality of life, and depression can also result. In addition to their mood altering abilities, cannabinoids have been shown to interact with the receptors in the spinal cord[25, 614, 636] and modulate inflammation and the pain response. Several studies have shown that cannabis has utility in the treatment of otherwise intractable pain from spinal cord damage.[211, 222, 277, 595, 635, 637, 638]

Additional Spasticity/spinal cord damage resources:
American Association of Neurological Surgeons: www.aans.org
American Stroke Association: www.strokeassociation.org
Christopher & Dana Reeve Foundation: www.christopherreeve.org
National Institute of Neurological Disorders and Stroke:
www.ninds.nih.gov
National Multiple Sclerosis Society: www.nationalmssociety.org
National Stroke Association:
www.stroke.org
Paralyzed Veterans of America:
www.pva.org

Spinocerebellar ataxia

Spinocerebellar ataxia is a condition in which part of the nervous system that controls movement is damaged. The condition causes a lack of muscle control in the arms and legs leading to lack of balance and coordination. With some types of ataxia, there may be speech and swallowing difficulties and dizziness. The National Institute of Neurological Disorders and Stroke indicates that ataxia refers to a set of symptoms or a family of disorders, but is not a specific diagnosis in and of itself. Ataxias can be hereditary and caused by genetic variants on different chromosomes; they can also be "sporadic", meaning that they have a genetic cause, but the genetic variant showed up newly in the patient, and was not in a parent. Ataxias can also be acquired and are common in stroke, multiple sclerosis, tumors, alcoholism, peripheral neuropathy, metabolic disorders, and vitamin deficiencies.

Cannabis has neuromodulatory and antispasmodic properties that can make it useful for patients with ataxia. See Tables 1 and 2 and sections on Muscle spasms; Multiple sclerosis; and Peripheral neuropathy for more information and references.

Additional Spinocerebellar ataxia resources:
National Ataxia Foundation: www.ataxia.org
National Institute of Neurological Disorders and Stroke:
www.ninds.nih.gov
Spinocerebellar Ataxia.org: spinocerebellerataxia.org

Tourette syndrome

Tourette syndrome is a neurological disorder characterized by involuntary movements that typically begin in the face, limbs, or trunk. The disorder is usually diagnosed in childhood and is more common in males than females. The US CDC indicates that 1 of every 360 children between the ages of 6 and 17 has been diagnosed with Tourette syndrome. The cause of Tourette syndrome is unknown, but it is thought that a complicated interaction of genetic influences and environmental factors are involved. Parents with Tourette syndrome have a 50% likelihood of passing the disease on to offspring, and in affected children, abnormal metabolism of dopamine in the brain can trigger the symptoms. Environmental risk factors that have been associated with Tourette's are fetal exposure to alcohol or tobacco smoke, birth complications and low birth weight, and certain streptococcal infections.

The main symptoms of Tourette syndrome are motor and vocal tics, defined by the US CDC as "sudden twitches, movements, or sounds that people do repeatedly" and that are uncontrollable. Motor tics are body movements such as blinking, shrugging, or jerking a limb. Vocal tics include humming, clearing the throat, or yelling out a word or phrase. Tics can also be simple and involve just a few body parts, or complex, with multiple body parts and a pattern to the movements. Tics are more pronounced when a person is under stress or excited. The US CDC reports that co-occurring conditions, especially attention deficit hyperactivity disorder and obsessive-compulsive disorder, are common and occur in some 86% of children diagnosed with Tourette syndrome.

There is no cure for Tourette syndrome, and some individuals with minimal symptoms do not require treatment. Medications can be used to treat severe or disruptive tics, as well as to reduce symptoms of co-occurring conditions. All of these medications have side effects, including weight gain, muscle stiffness, fatigue and restlessness. There are also behavioral therapies that can help patients reduce the frequency, severity, or impact of tics on their lives. A recent study of induced head twitch responses in mice indicated that activation of the CB1 receptors by enhancing endocannabinoid levels reduced head twitch in all strains.[640] This research supports prior clinical studies that found cannabis to significantly improve symptoms of tics,[641, 643, 644, 646, 647] and in some cases co-occurring obsessive compulsive disorder as well,[642] and there were no long-lasting adverse effects from the cannabis.[645]

Additional Tourette syndrome resources:
Jim Eisenreich Foundation for Children with Tourette Syndrome: www.tourettes.org
National Alliance for the Mentally Ill: www.nami.org
National Institute of Neurological Disorders and Stroke: www.ninds.nih.gov
National Tourette Syndrome Association: www.tsa-usa.org
Stuttering Foundation of America: www.stutteringhelp.org
Tourette Syndrome Foundation of Canada: www.tourette.ca
Tourette Syndrome "Plus": www.tourettesyndrome.net
US Centers for Disease Control and Prevention: www.cdc.gov

Traumatic brain injury

The US CDC indicates that traumatic brain injuries cause a significant number of deaths and permanent disability each year: they estimate that in 2010, about 2.5 million traumatic brain injuries occurred in the United States. About 5.3 million Americans are thought to be living with a disability related to a traumatic brain injury. Traumatic brain injury occurs when the normal function of the brain is interrupted by a blow or jolt to the head, or a penetrating head wound. The injury can range from mild to severe, as can the long-term outcomes of the injury.

A mild traumatic brain injury is also known as a concussion. The US CDC has a publication specifically about concussions entitled "Heads Up. Facts for Physicians about Mild Traumatic Brain Injury (MTBI" that can be found at www.cdc.gov/concussion/headsup/pdf/Facts_for_Physicians_booklet-a.pdf.

They indicate that the physical, cognitive, emotional and/or sleep-related symptoms of a concussion may last from several minutes to days, weeks, months, or even longer. After a concussion, the disturbance of brain function that occurs is not as much from structural injury or damage as it is to a change in brain metabolism. Four types of post-concussion signs/symptoms are listed:

- *Physical* symptoms include headache, nausea and vomiting, balance difficulty, dizziness, visual problems, fatigue, light and sound sensitivity, numbness/tingling, and dazed or stunned feeling

- *Cognitive* symptoms include mental "fog", feeling slowed down, concentration and memory difficulties, confusion about recent events, repeating questions or answering questions slowly

- *Emotional* symptoms include irritability, sadness, anxiety, excess emotionality

- *Sleep* symptoms include drowsiness, sleeping more or less than usual, trouble falling asleep

These symptoms typically resolve within a month, but sometimes can persist up to years, or even permanently and cause disability – this is known as post-concussion syndrome (PCS).[666]

People who suffer severe traumatic brain injuries are likely to be hospitalized, and 43% of those are estimated to experience a short- or long-term disability that can affect attention and memory, motor function, sensation, and emotion. Brain injury can also occur from insufficient blood flow to the brain (termed brain ischemia, cerebral ischemia, or cerebrovascular ischemia). Irreversible brain injury can occur if blood flow is interrupted for more than a few minutes, and symptoms can be similar to those in individuals who suffered a traumatic brain injury.

In a study of ischemic brain injury in a mouse model,[50] cannabis compound CBD prevented tissue death and improved neurological condition and motor function. These findings are similar to those of Kwiatkoski[635] in rats that experienced spinal cord injury. This may be due to activation of the CB2 receptors, as a study of induced traumatic brain injury in mice determined that activation of these receptors was associated with recovery of motor and exploratory function.[648] In a large study of humans who sustained traumatic brain injuries, the compound THC was also found to be significantly associated with increased survival.[297] A study of patients with minor traumatic brain injury that focused upon factors that might diminish neural reserve (and thus increase post-traumatic amnesia) found that pre-injury cannabis use did not diminish neural reserve.[649]

> Additional Traumatic brain injury resources:
> Alzheimer's Association: www.alz.org
> American Speech-Language-Hearing Association: www.asha.org
> Brain Injury Association of America: www.biausa.org
> Brain Injury Resource Center: www.headinjury.com
> Brainline.org: www.brainline.org
> Center of Excellence for Medical Multimedia:
> www.traumaticbraininjuryatoz.org
> National Institute of Neurological Disorders and Stroke:
> www.ninds.nih.gov
> The Brain Trauma Foundation: www.braintrauma.org
> Traumatic.Brain.Injury.Com: www.traumaticbraininjury.com
> US Centers for Disease Control and Prevention: www.cdc.gov

Treatment with AZT, chemotherapy, protease inhibitors, radiotherapy

Serious conditions such as cancers and HIV/AIDS require medical treatments that typically cause debilitating side effects. Some of these side effects are temporary and some are minor, but others are long lasting and/or severe and life-threatening. Even seemingly minor side effects such as fatigue and nausea can adversely impact a patient's ability to perform daily functions, and many side effects make holding down a job, going to school, or even having a social life difficult to impossible. Sometimes side effects are so troubling that patients do not comply fully with their treatment regimen, and sometimes they even decide to discontinue treatment altogether.. Research since the 1970s has shown that cannabis can help ease side effects of medical treatments, and help patients comply with treatment regimens.[654, 655] Below are summarized some of the major side effects and scientific references for the known benefits of cannabis for easing symptoms. Additional information about the effects of cannabis on nausea, pain, peripheral neuropathy, spasticity, and vomiting, can be found in the respective sections of this manual.

The American Cancer Society (www.cancer.org) provides a detailed list of treatment types and their known side effects, which are divided into physical and emotional effects. Most typical are pain, nausea and vomiting, fatigue, anemia, lymphedema, infections, fertility and sexual side effects, incontinence, loss of appetite, "chemo brain", peripheral neuropathy, and hearing and motor problems. One widely used chemotherapy agent, doxorubicin, has limited clinical application because of its dose-dependent toxicity to the heart. A recent study in a mouse model of doxorubicin-induced cardiomyopathy showed that CBD can affect cellular organelles known as mitochondria in a manner that protects against doxorubicin damage.[49] AIDS info at the National Health Institutes (aidsinfo.nih.gov) discusses in detail some of the major known side effects of antiretroviral treatments, including hepatotoxicity, hyperglycemia, hyperlipidemia, lactic acidosis, lipodystrophy, osteonecrosis, osteoporosis, osteopenia, and skin rash. Each of these major side effects has its own set of symptoms, briefly described below. A common theme of most of these therapy-induced conditions is the prevalence of nausea and vomiting. Systematic literature reviews and clinical trials have found that orally-administered cannabinoids and/or smoked cannabis, [120, 128, 130, 132, 136, 140, 153, 156, 157, 161, 166, 168, 176, 177, 182, 183, 254, 261, 262, 650–653] as well as synthetic cannabinoids[255] are as effective, or even more effective, than conventional drugs at reducing nausea and vomiting. Additionally, cannabinoids are excellent appetite stimulants for individuals who suffer anorexia due to illness or treatment.[174] Mood problems, particularly depression, also occur commonly with debilitating diseases, and as side effects of treatments.[174]

- *Hepatotoxicity* is a broad term to describe damage to the liver: hepatitis (see Hepatitis C), death of liver cells, and fatty liver. Symptoms of hepatotoxicity include nausea, vomiting, abdominal pain, anorexia, diarrhea, fatigue, yellowing of the skin and eyes, and enlarged liver.

Three classes of anti-HIV medications can cause hepatotoxicity: non-nucleoside reverse transcriptase inhibitors (NNRTIs), nucleoside reverse transcriptase inhibitors (NRTIs), and protease inhibitors (PIs). Hepatotoxicity is sufficiently serious that in most cases, medications must be stopped or changed. In an animal model of induced hepato- toxicity,[45] cannabidiol significantly ameliorated liver tissue injury.

- *Hyperglycemia* means that there is too much glucose (a type of sugar) in the blood. HIV protease inhibitors can cause hyperglycemia, particularly in people who are older, overweight, or have a familial history of diabe- tes. Symptoms of hyperglycemia include increased urination, excessive hunger or thirst, and unexplained weight loss. Treatment for hypergly- cemia can include medications or insulin to decrease blood sugar lev- els, or in some cases, discontinuation of the protease inhibitors.

- *Hyperlipidemia* means that there is too much fat in the blood, a condi- tion that can lead to heart disease and pancreatitis (see Pancreatitis). Either fortunately or unfortunately, depending upon how you view it, hyperlipidemia has no overt symptoms: laboratory tests must be per- formed to monitor blood levels at least once per year. Hyperlipidemia can be caused by protease inhibitors. Treatments for hyperlipidemia include weight and diet control, exercise, smoking and alcohol cessa- tion or limitation, and maintenance of blood pressure. There are also medications that can lower fats in the blood, but these also have side effects including nausea, vomiting, and more serious side effects. In some cases, hyperlipidemia may be severe or refractory to treatment, and anti-HIV medications may need to be changed or discontinued.

- *Lactic acidosis* is characterized by too much lactate (which comes from lactic acid, which is produced when the body produces energy) and too much acid in the blood. Lactic acidosis can be associated with fatty liver. It is a serious and life-threatening condition that can indicate the body is making too much lactate, or that the liver is unable to break the lactate down. Lactic acidosis can be caused by NRTIs, and women, overweight people, and people taking certain medications may be at increased risk for the condition. Symptoms of lactic acidosis are nau- sea, vomiting and abdominal pain, fatigue, shortness of breath, rapid breathing, enlarged or tender liver, cold or blue extremities, abnormal heart beat, and weight loss. Treatment for lactic acidosis involves cessation of NRTI medications, hospitalization, and sometimes administration of intravenous fluids and breathing assistance.

- *Lipodystrophy* is also called fat redistribution, and comes in two forms: fat wasting and fat accumulation. Fat wasting is where fat is lost from arms, legs, face and buttocks, while fat accumulation is buildup of fat in the belly, breasts, and back of the neck. Lipodystrophy is thought to be caused by taking a combination of NRTIs and PIs simultaneously. Older people, people of European origin, people who have longer and more severe HIV infection, and obese people are at increased risk for lipodystrophy. Also, sex influences how lipodystrophy is experienced, with men being more likely to have fat wasting in the arms and legs, and women more likely to have fat accumulation in abdomen and breasts. Treatments for lipodystrophy are not entirely effective, but include changes to anti-HIV medications, diet and exercise control, certain medications, and injections, implants, and surgery to remove fat accumulation.

- *Osteonecrosis* is death of the bone, which occurs when the blood supply is cut off to areas of the bone. It is unclear if osteonecrosis occurs because of medication side effects, or due directly to the HIV infection. Symptoms of osteonecrosis include pain, limited range of motion, joint stiffness, muscle spasms, and damage leading to bone collapse. Treatment of osteonecrosis includes medications for pain relief and surgery to remove the dead bone and replace the joint.

- *Osteopenia* and *osteoporosis* are conditions in which the bones lose calcium and phosphate and thus lose density; osteoporosis is the more severe form of osteopenia. Osteopenia and osteoporosis can be caused by PIs, and females, smokers, individuals of low body weight, and those who take certain medications or drink excessive amounts of alcohol may be of increased risk. Osteopenia andosteoporosis have no obvious symptoms until bone loss is sufficient that fractures occur, typically in the spine, wrists, or hips. These fractures result in pain or tenderness, loss of height, and stooped posture.

- *Skin rashes* are something that everyone has experienced at some time or another, but any of the three main anti-HIV medications can cause mild and severe, life-threatening rashes. Two types of severe skin rash are Stevens-Johnson syndrome (SJS) and toxic epidermal necrolysis (TEN). Both are the same type of skin rash, but TEN involves a much more extensive amount of skin—at least 30% of total body skin area. Symptoms of SJS and TEN include skin spots that develop central blisters, blisters of the mouth, eyes, or genitalia, peeling skin with painful sores, fever, headache, and general malaise. These types of rashes are severe and require either a change of medication or an antihistamine medication along with the anti-HIV medications. A potentially life-threatening rash that occurs with the DRESS syndrome (drug rash with eosinophilia and systemic symptoms) causes whole body symptoms such as fever, blood abnormalities, and inflammation of organs. Severe SJS, TEN, or DRESS can require cessation of anti-HIV medications, hospital admittance, and administration of intravenous fluids and anti-inflammatory and antibiotic medications. In cases of TEN with severe skin loss, the person may even need to be admitted to a burn unit. Research in a mouse models indicates that topically applied cannabinoids are effective at decreasing allergic inflammation, and may hold potential for treating inflammatory skin conditions.[141, 268]

Vomiting: intractable (see also Nausea)

Nausea and vomiting are common responses to conditions such as pregnancy, motion sickness, and extreme emotions such as fear and anxiety, but they can also be induced by certain medications and radiation therapy. In addition to the scientific studies discussed in the sections on Nausea and on Treatment with AZT, chemotherapy, protease inhibitors, radiotherapy, several studies have found cannabinoids to be efficient at ameliorating vomiting in animal models.[79, 85, 114, 134, 657]

TABLE 4. Approved conditions, effects (beneficial, no significant change/negative evaluation, detrimental) and scientific references*

CONDITION	BENEFICIAL	NEUTRAL	DETRIMENTAL
Acquired immune deficiency syndrome (AIDS)	119, 205, 286, 291, 292, 305, 473–478	479, 480	481
Alzheimer's disease	22, 44, 69, 90, 138, 482–484		
Amyotrophic lateral sclerosis (ALS)	22, 249, 294, 300, 485–488		
Anorexia	301, 302, 305, 306, 474, 483, 489–493	178	494
Arnold-Chiari malformation (see Pain: chronic; Nausea; Migraine)			
Arthritis	39, 67, 208, 229, 234, 348, 495–501		
Cancer	16, 27, 51, 54, 64, 68, 70, 82, 87, 91, 94, 104, 105, 110, 112, 122–126, 142, 143, 146, 155, 158, 160, 172, 175, 185, 188, 217, 269–272, 274, 275, 313, 334, 502–512	513–515	93, 334–337, 339–343
Cachexia	118, 303, 516–518	178, 494	
Causalgia (see Pain: chronic/severe/ intractable)			
Chronic inflammatory demyelinating polyneuropathy (CIPD) (see Peripheral neuropathy)			
Chronic renal failure	46		
Cirrhosis	15, 76, 519	520	364–366
Crohn's disease	238, 307, 490, 521–523		238
Dystonia	38, 253, 524–527		
Epilepsy	42, 57, 244, 246–248, 527–534	535	404
Fibromyalgia	197, 220, 229, 536		
Fibrous dysplasia (see Pain: chronic/severe/ intractable)			
Glaucoma	137, 181, 263, 265–267, 537–546		
Hepatitis C	489, 547	520, 548	365–367, 549
Hospice/terminal illness	550, 551		

*Scientific references are located at the end of the book following the glossary, in numerical order.

(Continued)

TABLE 4. *(Continued)*

CONDITION	BENEFICIAL	NEUTRAL	DETRIMENTAL
Human immunodeficiency virus (HIV) infection	119, 127, 205, 286, 291, 292, 305, 474, 477, 478, 493, 552	479	93
Huntington's disease	88, 553–556	557	
Hydrocephalus (see Migraine; Nausea; Seizures; Vomiting: intractable)			
Inflammatory bowel disease (IBD)	28, 31, 56, 111, 238, 490, 523, 558, 559		
Interstitial cystitis (see Pain: chronic/severe/ intractable)			
Lupus (see Arthritis)			
Migraine	197, 478, 560–567		
Multiple sclerosis (MS)	22, 58, 59, 71, 72, 77, 151, 184, 210, 214, 216, 225, 232, 235, 276, 278, 279, 281–285, 293, 298, 299, 476, 491, 500, 552, 568–593	338	344–346, 375, 376
Muscle spasms	171, 232, 276, 282, 284, 285, 491, 500, 569, 570, 578, 582, 588, 594, 595		
Muscular dystrophy (see Spasticity; Pain: chronic/severe/ intractable; Chapter 4 Anxiety)			
Myasthenia gravis (see Chapter 4 Anxiety disorders; Autoimmune disorders)			
Myoclonus (see Muscle spasms; Seizures)			
Nail patella syndrome (see Arthritis; Glaucoma; Pain: chronic/severe/ intractable)			
Nausea	86, 102, 103, 162, 169, 170, 179, 182, 256–259, 261, 489, 547, 558, 596–600		
Neurofibromatosis (see Cancer; Migraine; Pain: chronic/severe/ intractable; Peripheral neuropathy; Seizures)	285		

*Scientific references are located at the end of the book following the glossary, in numerical order.

(Continued)

TABLE 4. *(Continued)*

CONDITION	BENEFICIAL	NEUTRAL	DETRIMENTAL
Pain: chronic/severe/ intractable	25, 40, 77, 95, 96, 98, 147, 154, 204–206, 208, 209, 215–218, 221, 222, 224–226, 228–231, 235–242, 259, 285, 478, 491, 493, 500, 506, 558, 569, 572, 574, 593, 601–620	165, 595, 621	
Pancreatitis	622		399–403
Parkinson's disease	33, 35, 61, 191, 227, 623	624, 625	
Peripheral neuropathy	40, 80, 205, 207, 212, 213, 218, 225, 233, 241, 242, 608, 626	237	237
Post-traumatic stress disorder (PTSD)	30, 288, 627–630		
Rheumatoid arthritis (see Arthritis)			
Seizures	32, 36, 37, 42, 57, 106, 135, 180, 186, 187, 244–248, 528–533, 631–634	535	404–408, 472
Sjögren's syndrome (see Arthritis; Chapter 4 Autoimmune disorders)			
Spasticity/spinal cord damage	25, 171, 211, 222, 232, 276, 277, 280, 282, 284, 285, 491, 500, 569, 570, 578, 582, 588, 593–595, 614, 635–638		639
Spinocerebellar ataxia (see Muscle spasms; Multiple sclerosis; Peripheral neuropathy)			
Tourette syndrome	640–647		
Traumatic brain injury	50, 297, 635, 648	649	
Treatment with AZT, chemotherapy, protease inhibitors, radiotherapy	45, 49, 120, 128, 130, 133, 136, 140, 141, 153, 156, 157, 161, 162, 166, 168, 174, 176, 177, 179, 182, 183, 254, 255, 258, 261, 262, 477, 498, 596, 600, 608, 609, 622, 650–655	129, 656	
Vomiting: intractable	60, 79, 85, 114, 120, 134, 162, 169, 170, 179, 182, 255, 259, 261, 596, 598, 600, 653, 657, 658		358–363

*Scientific references are located at the end of the book following the glossary, in numerical order.

(Continued)

CHAPTER 4

OTHER CONDITIONS FOR WHICH MARIJUANA MAY BE BENEFICIAL

As society begins to accept the possibility of cannabis-based medicines, scientific research into the conditions that cannabis can benefit continues. The following table provides a list of conditions for which there is at least one published scientific study that finds a beneficial effect of cannabis. As might be expected, for several of these conditions there are also other studies that found either no effect of cannabis, or that found a detrimental effect.

TABLE 5. Other non-approved conditions, effects (beneficial, no significant change/negative evaluation, detrimental) and scientific references*

CONDITION	BENEFICIAL	NEUTRAL	DETRIMENTAL
Acne vulgaris	78		667
Alcohol dependence	8, 201, 203		357
Anxiety disorders	29, 33, 41, 53, 73, 92, 139, 144, 287, 288, 319, 409, 478, 493, 502, 529, 617, 668–670	250, 671– 674	131, 316–318, 320–332, 471, 675
Asthma	159, 676–678		464, 465
Atherosclerosis	679–681		

*Scientific references are located at the end of the book following the glossary, in numerical order.

(Continued)

TABLE 5. *(Continued)*

CONDITION	BENEFICIAL	NEUTRAL	DETRIMENTAL
Atopic dermatitis	682		
Attention deficit hyperactivity disorder (ADD/ADHD)	683–685		
Autoimmune disorders	54, 58, 59, 659		
Bacterial infections: antibiotic resistant	12, 20		
Bipolar disorder	686–689	219, 690	251, 333, 388–394
Bladder dysfunction	210, 575, 581, 592		
Brachial plexus avulsion	207, 500		
Cerebral malaria	43		
Cerebral palsy	171, 248		
Chronic liver disease	15, 66, 489, 547	691	366–368
Chronic obstructive pulmonary disease (COPD)	692	693–695	466–469
Cocaine dependence	148, 200, 683, 696, 697		
Cystic fibrosis	23		470
Degenerative disc disease	698		
Depression	99, 117, 287, 333, 478, 493, 617, 699–701	409–411, 671, 672, 690, 702–712	261, 319, 329, 332, 348–357
Diabetes	81, 97, 113, 212, 311, 312, 713, 714	237	
Diarrhea	238, 252, 359, 490, 523, 558		283, 599, 715, 716
Herpes virus infection	163		371–374

*Scientific references are located at the end of the book following the glossary, in numerical order.

(Continued)

TABLE 5. *(Continued)*

CONDITION	BENEFICIAL	NEUTRAL	DETRIMENTAL
Hiccups: intractable	717		
Hypertension	121, 189, 264, 265, 718	719	370, 720
Night vision	193, 721		
Nystagmus	589, 722		395
Obesity	192, 308–311, 313, 723, 724		314, 315
Opioid dependence	83, 148–150, 199, 202, 683, 725	533, 726–730	396–398
Pain: acute	145, 223, 619	731, 732	369
Prostatitis: chronic	618		
Psoriasis	733		
Schizophrenia	47, 48, 52, 55, 62, 63, 65, 101, 208, 296, 734–757	100, 758–782	75, 317, 323, 333, 347, 377–387, 409–463, 672, 687, 783–808
Sickle cell disease	615	809	
Sleep disorders	33, 34, 53, 167, 227, 239, 474, 478, 500, 529, 593, 605, 617, 618, 630, 665, 810–817		
Transmissible spongiform encephalopathies (prion disease)	24		

Acne vulgaris

Acne, also known as acne vulgaris, is a skin condition most common in teenagers, but it can occur in anyone of any age. Acne is caused when the pores become clogged when the sebaceous glands produce too much oil. As the pore becomes blocked, dirt, bacteria, and cells build up, resulting in bumps and sometimes swelling. According to the National Library of Medicine, hormonal changes, certain cosmetic and hair products, heavy sweating and humidity, and drugs such as testosterone, estrogen, and phenytoin can trigger acne. Diets high in refined sugars or dairy products are also thought to be related to acne in some cases. Treatment for acne includes gentle daily cleansing of the skin and hair, avoidance of oily cosmetics, and medications that kill bacteria, dry skin oils, or peel the top layer of skin. There are also laser treatments, skin peels, dermabrasion removal of scars, or removal, drainage, or injection of acne cysts with cortisone.

Although the National Library of Medicine indicates that research has shown that chocolate, nuts, and greasy foods probably do not cause acne, a survey study of French individuals between ages 15 and 24 revealed people who consumed chocolate and sweets were 2.38 times more likely than those who did not to suffer acne, while people who smoked more than 10 cigarettes per day were less likely to have acne.[667] This study also found that regular cannabis smoking was associated with a higher likelihood of acne, however, this is in contrast to a study of the effects of cannabis that demonstrated that administration of CBD to cultured skin and sebocytes (the cells that produce oil) inhibited inflammation, and inhibited production of oil, suggesting CBD as a therapeutic agent for treatment of acne.[78]

Additional Acne vulgaris resources:
Acne.org: www.acne.org
American Academy of Dermatology: www.aad.org
National Library of Medicine:
www.ncbi.nlm.nih.gov

Alcohol dependence

Alcohol dependence, or alcoholism, is a chronic disease that includes the following four characteristics, as defined by the National Council on Alcoholism and Drug Dependence: craving for alcohol, loss of control, physical dependence that includes withdrawal symptoms after drinking cessation, and tolerance for alcohol. In the United States, 1 in every 12 adults is estimated to suffer from alcohol abuse or alcohol dependence. Alcohol abuse is different from alcohol dependence in that alcohol abusers have some ability to set limits on their drinking, but alcohol abuse is still dangerous. Alcoholics need more alcohol over time to feel the same effect, have withdrawal symptoms when alcohol wears off, lose control when they drink, neglect other activities, and may want to stop drinking but be unable to. Alcoholism is harmful to the drinker, because heavy chronic drinking contributes to liver disease, cardiovascular diseases, pancreatitis, a depressed immune system and consequently to susceptibility to infectious diseases and cancers, hormonal deficiencies, sexual dysfunction and infertility, early menopause and menstrual irregularities. Alcohol is also harmful to families and to society. Alcoholism is associated with increase in divorce and separations, in domestic violence, in traffic injuries and fatalities, and in other types of accidents. Additionally, pregnant women who drink may give birth to a child with fetal alcohol syndrome.

A 1970 case study of an alcoholic patient found that cannabis helped reduction of alcohol consumption.[201] The patient is quoted comparing marijuana to alcohol, "it made me high like alcohol, but it didn't give me that feeling in the pit of my stomach when I felt *angry*." The study's author concludes that cannabis contributed a sense of euphoria and detachment similar to alcohol, but lacked several of the negative psychological effects, and warrants further clinical trial in treatment of alcoholism. In a survey study focused on harm reduction (defined as "a treatment approach that seeks to minimize the occurrence of drug/alcohol addiction and its impacts on the addict/alcoholic and society at large") among alcohol abusers and others with conditions prohibiting alcohol,[8] inhaled cannabis was used to reduce alcohol consumption. Perceived effects of cannabis that allowed cessation or reduction of alcohol consumption included relaxation, pain relief, and sleep benefits. Another anonymous survey of 350 medical cannabis patients in California found that 40% used cannabis as a substitute for alcohol, 26% as a substitute for illicit drugs, and 66% as a substitute for prescription drugs.[203] Most common reasons for substituting cannabis were fewer adverse side effects, better symptom management, and less withdrawal potential. Clearly, cannabis may be of utility in helping some patients reduce their dependence on alcohol.

Additional Alcohol dependence resources:
Alcoholics Anonymous: www.aa.org
Drinkaware.co.uk:
www.drinkaware.co.uk
National Council on Alcoholism and Drug Dependence: ncadd.org
National Institute on Alcohol Abuse and Alcoholism: www.niaaa.nih.
gov

Anxiety disorders

Anxiety disorders are a common form of emotional disorder, causing a person to be fearful and uncertain, and leading them to avoid situations that might make them more anxious. An anxiety disorder differs from normal anxiety caused by a particular situation in that an anxiety disorder lasts at least 6 months, and can get worse if not treated. The National Institute of Mental Health indicates that every year anxiety disorders affect about 40 million US adults over 18 years of age. Anxiety disorders commonly co-occur with other mental illnesses or physical illnesses. The American Psychiatric Association describes the common symptoms of anxiety disorders as overwhelming feelings of panic/fear, uncontrollable obsessive thoughts, painful intrusive memories, recurring nightmares, and physical symptoms such as nausea, heart pounding, muscle tension, and easily startling. They list three major types of anxiety disorder: Panic Disorder, Phobias, and Generalized Anxiety Disorder, and there is an additional anxiety disorder called Obsessive-Compulsive Disorder.

- *Panic Disorder* is characterized by panic attacks, which are overwhelming, frightening, and distressing. Symptoms include pounding heart or chest pain, sweating, trembling, or shaking, shortness of breath or a feeling of choking, nausea or abdominal pain, dizziness, feeling disconnected or unreal, fear of losing control, dying, or going crazy, numbness, and chills or hot flashes. People having a panic attack often believe they are on the brink of death. People with panic disorder will go to great lengths to avoid situations that they believe may precipitate future panic attacks.

- *Phobias* are defined by the American Psychiatric Association as "an excessive and persistent fear of a specific object, situation, or activity." As with patients with panic disorder, people with phobias may go to great lengths to avoid what they fear. The fear may be of a specific object (like spiders) or of situations (like air travel), of a social or performance situation (known as social anxiety disorder), or of being where they cannot escape or cannot be helped if they panic (known as agoraphobia). Some people with agoraphobia cannot leave their home.

- *Generalized anxiety disorders* are characterized by ongoing tension of a severity that interferes with daily functioning. Common symptoms are sleeping problems, muscle aches and tension, nausea, weakness, headaches, irritability, and difficulty concentrating.

- *Obsessive-compulsive disorder* (OCD) is characterized by frequent, upsetting thoughts or fears, and/or needs to perform certain routines/rituals over and over – these are called obsessions. Obsessions differ from the normal preoccupations that healthy people might have, in that obsessions cause distress to the person, and they interfere with daily life. The person does not get pleasure from performing the obsessive ritual or behavior, but they do get relief from the anxiety that is caused if they do not perform the behavior. The National Institute of Mental Health indicates that OCD affects about 2.2 million US adults, and usually begins in childhood, adolescence, or early adulthood. The disease may be accompanied by eating disorders, other anxiety disorders, or depression.

The National Institute of Mental Health indicates that, although the exact causes of anxiety disorders are unknown, they are complex and research indicates that a combination of genetics and environmental stresses are probably involved. Two parts of the brain appear to be key in anxiety disorders: the amygdala and the hippocampus. The amygdala seems to process incoming signals from the senses, and is responsible for alerting the brain if a threat is present, triggering fear or anxiety responses. Emotional memories seem to be stored in the amygdala. The hippocampus is responsible for turning threatening events into memories, and it may be involved in flashbacks that are part of post-traumatic stress disorder (discussed in Chapter 3). Two types of treatment available for anxiety disorders are psychotherapy (also known as talk therapy) and medications. People often use a combination of the two, although medications may have side effects.

Several laboratory studies on animal models of stress and anxiety have been performed. In an attempt to determine the manner in which cannabis decreases anxiety, the benzodiazepine receptor was examined in mice;[668] chronic treatment with cannabis appeared to "prime" the receptors, causing increased affinity and reduction in anxiety. Acute treatment with cannabis, on the other hand, had no effect on anxiety. In stressed animals, high doses of THC can reduce stress, while low doses have the opposite effect and increase stress.[139] In animals that were not previously stressed, both low and high doses of THC had an anxiolytic (anxiety reducing) effect. A study of cannabidiol on stressed animals indicated that it reduced anxiety.[73] Cannabidiol injected into the amygdala of an anxiety-induced sleep-disturbed rat model produced anxiety reduction in rapid-eye movement sleep.[53] Repeated administration of CBD in rats also induces anti-panic effects, probably by acting on the 5-HT1A serotonin receptors.[29, 92]

In healthy cannabis users, THC reduces the reactivity of the amygdala to threat signals, decreasing anxiety.[144, 669] A consistent result was found in patients with both major depression and cannabis dependence, wherein a higher level of smoked cannabis use was also associated with lower amygdala reactivity.[287] In patients with social anxiety disorder, cannabidiol had significant anxiolytic effects compared to patients receiving a placebo.[818] Cannabidiol also reduced frequency of obsessive-compulsive behaviors.[670] Several studies have found a significant association between anxiety disorders and cannabis use,[318, 325] although the results of other research studies indicate that this relationship could be due to the anxiolytic effects of cannabis, or cannabis could precipitate anxiety in vulnerable individuals.[329] This may be due to the different effects of THC and CBD on the body, with THC more likely to induce anxiety, dysphoria, positive psychotic symptoms, physical and mental sedation, subjective intoxication, and increased heart rate, while CBD had none of these effects.[327] A study of 100 young adults indicated that, although the most frequently reported effect of cannabis use was relaxation, as many as 40% reported paranoid feelings, with heavier usage being associated with the paranoia.[409] There are other reports of cannabis use increasing anxiety or even precipitating panic attacks,[317, 320, 330] particularly in adolescents,[316, 321, 332] although a large study of 1709 adolescents found that, after controlling for the effects of daily cigarette smoking, cannabis was not associated with the development of panic.[673] Occasional use of cannabis among anxiety and depression outpatients also did not associate with panic disorder or social phobia symptoms.[250] Studies in which cannabinoids have been isolated and administered individually show that THC can trigger anxiety, worry, depression, negative self-thoughts, and lead to acute paranoia in vulnerable individuals.[131, 322, 323, 326] An additional study showed that, while not all individuals who used cannabis experienced heightened anxiety or depression, among those who did experience these negative outcomes, a higher dose of cannabis was associated with higher anxiety scores.[324] In laboratory situations, intravenously administered THC has also been associated with schizophrenia-like and other undesirable symptoms.[415, 471, 675]

Additional Anxiety disorder resources:
American Psychiatric Association:
www.psychiatry.org
National Institute of Mental Health: www.nimh.nih.gov

Asthma

Asthma is a chronic, potentially life-threatening, disease of the lungs. An asthma attack is triggered when certain things in the environment, such as weather conditions, dust, chemicals, smoke, pet dander, or mold cause the airways that lead to the lungs to become inflamed. Inflammation of the airways leads to extra mucus formation and more swelling, which then makes breathing very difficult. The person ends up with chest tightness, wheezing, and breathlessness. Asthma affects people of all ages, and the US CDC estimates that it affects 25.7 million people in the US. The condition can be serious, and in 2010 about 1.8 million people are reported to have visited an emergency room for asthma-related care.

Asthma is treated by avoiding asthma triggers and by taking medications. A laboratory guinea pig study examined the efficacy of THC, CBD,

CBG, CBC, THCV, and cannabidiolic acid on the airway hyperresponsiveness, airway inflammation, and cough and found that THC was able to act favorably upon each of these through activation of the CB1 and CB2 receptors.[159] A study by Tashkin and colleagues in 1974[676] sought to verify the nineteenth century purported uses of cannabis to treat asthma. They treated human subjects who had asthma either with a placebo, with smoked marijuana, or with orally administered THC and measured their airway resistance and conductance. They found that both the smoked marijuana and the oral THC caused bronchodilation (opening of the airways) for at least 2 hours. They also found that smoked marijuana was able to reverse experimentally induced asthma in human subjects.[243] It is important to note, however, that in people who are allergic to cannabis, it can also stimulate an asthma attack,[465] and smoking marijuana may also have the same adverse respiratory effects as smoking tobacco (e.g., chronic bronchitis, coughing, wheezing, phlegm production).[464]

Additional Asthma resources:
Allergy & Asthma Network:
www.aanma.org
American Academy of Allergy, Asthma, and Immunology: www.aaaai.org
American College of Allergy, Asthma and Immunology: www.acaai.org
American Lung Association:
www.lung.org
Asthma and Allergy Foundation of America: www.aafa.org
National Heart, Lung, and Blood Institute: www.nhlbi.nih.gov
US Centers for Disease Control and Prevention: www.cdc.gov
World Health Organization:
www.who.int

Atherosclerosis

Arteriosclerotic heart disease occurs when the arteries become stiffened and cannot properly transmit oxygen and nutrients from the heart to the rest of the body. Arteriosclerosis is also known as hardening of the arteries. A specific and common type of arteriosclerosis is atherosclerosis, in which fat, cholesterol, and other substances cause deposits known as "plaques" to build up on the walls of arteries, ultimately blocking the flow of blood. Atherosclerosis is associated with aging, but high levels of cholesterol in the blood can also cause the condition at younger ages. Risk factors include alcohol use, lack of exercise, overweight condition, and a diet too high in certain types of fats. When tissues and organs are starved of blood and oxygen they become damaged or even die; atherosclerosis is a common cause of heart attack and stroke. The National Heart, Lung, and Blood Institute lists several types of treatment for atherosclerosis, including lifestyle changes such as smoking cessation, alcohol and fatty food limitation, and regular physical activity. In some cases, medications may be prescribed for high blood pressure or for high cholesterol levels if lifestyle changes are insufficient to address the problem. Atherosclerosis is preventable, and although it is not reversible once it has occurred, lifestyle changes and medication may be able to slow the process once it has begun, reducing the chances of heart attack and stroke.

Laboratory research on cannabinoids isolated from *Cannabis sativa* have been shown to reduce the formation of cholesterol in cultured human cells by making it unavailable for the cell's metabolic processes.[681] THC was also shown to inhibit an enzyme called 15-LOX that is an important component of atherosclerosis.[680] In a mouse model of atherosclerosis, daily oral administration of THC significantly inhibited progression of the disease by acting at the CB2 receptors.[679]

Additional Atherosclerosis resources:
American Heart Association:
www.heart.org
National Heart, Lung and Blood Institute: www.nhlbi.nih.gov
US Centers for Disease Control and Prevention: www.cdc.gov

Atopic dermatitis

Atopic dermatitis is a common skin disease also known as "eczema". It is very common in children, and the American Academy of Dermatology indicates that about 10-20% of all children in the world have atopic dermatitis. Although it can occur in adults as well, it almost always begins in childhood. Atopic dermatitis is more common today than even 30 years ago, for unclear reasons. It is not contagious. Risk factors include having a family member with atopic dermatitis, hay fever, or asthma, living in a developed country or cold climate, being part of a higher social class, and being born to an older mother. Symptoms of atopic dermatitis are different depending upon the age of the person, but generally there is an itchy, dry rash, potentially with scaly patches and thickening of the skin. Atopic dermatitis can lead to skin infections. There is no cure for atopic dermatitis, but it can be treated by lifestyle changes, medications, and skin care. A study of atopic dermatitis in human subjects in 2005 found that dietary hempseed oil (which comes from cannabis) was able to improve symptoms of dryness and itchiness.[682]

Additional Atopic dermatitis resources:
American Academy of Dermatology: www.aad.org
National Eczema Association: nationaleczema.org
National Institute of Arthritis and Musculoskeletal and Skin Diseases: www.niams.nih.gov

Attention deficit hyperactivity disorder (ADD/ADHD)

Attention deficit hyperactivity disorder is often referred to simply as "ADHD". It is a condition in which normal childhood behaviors of inattentiveness, hyperactivity, or impulsiveness are exaggerated and excessive. The National Institute of Mental Health (NIMH) indicates that ADHD is one of the most common childhood disorders, boys are four times more likely than girls to have it, and about 9% of American children age 13 to 18 years of age are affected. The disorder can continue into adulthood. In order for a child to be diagnosed with ADHD, symptoms must occur for at least 6 months and occur to a greater degree than that seen in other children of the same age. NIMH provides a long list of symptoms/behaviors, just a few of which are repeated here:

- *Inattention*: easily distracted, difficulty focusing on one thing, trouble completing or turning in homework assignments, daydreaming, becoming easily confused, difficulty following instructions.

- *Hyperactivity*: fidgeting, nonstop talking, difficulty sitting still, constant motion, difficulty doing quiet activities.

- *Impulsivity*: impatience, interrupting conversations/activities of others, difficulty waiting.

Other conditions may co-occur with ADHD, for example a learning disability, anxiety and depression, bipolar disorder, Tourette syndrome, sleep disorders, and substance use disorders. The causes of ADHD are not entirely known, but genetics appear to be important along with other environmental factors. There is no cure for ADHD, but there are treatments to reduce the symptoms and help the person to function. Treatments include medication, psychotherapy, education, and training. Medications most commonly used for ADHD are stimulants, which actually calm people with the condition. These medications have side effects, however, such as decreased appetite, sleep problems, anxiety, irritability, and development of sudden, repetitive movements or sounds (also known as "tics").

Analysis of a large sample (4117 individuals) of marijuana users in California found that a significant portion of applicants had been diagnosed with ADHD as children, and inhaled small amounts of cannabis to enhance concentration abilities and reduce anxiety.[684] In a study of outpatients being treated for both cocaine dependence and ADHD, moderate cannabis use was associated with better treatment outcome (abstinence from cocaine) compared to no, minimal, or heavy cannabis users.[683]

Additional Attention deficit hyperactivity disorder resources:
American Psychological Association: apa.org
American Speech-Language-Hearing Association: www.asha.org
Children and Adults with Attention-Deficit/Hyperactivity Disorder (CHADD): www.chadd.org
National Alliance for the Mentally Ill: www.nami.org
National Institute of Mental Health: www.nimh.nih.gov
National Resource Center on AD/HD: www.help4adhd.org

Autoimmune disorders

Autoimmune disorders are those in which the body's own immune system mistakenly attacks healthy body tissues. Normally, the immune system helps to protect the body from bacteria, viruses, cancer cells, toxins, and other foreign substances. In an autoimmune disorder, the immune system cannot tell the difference between healthy body tissue and foreign substances or diseased tissues. The National Library of Medicine indicates that there are more than 80 types of autoimmune disorders. The causes of autoimmune disorders are unknown, but are thought to be a combination of genetic predisposition and environmental factors that may trigger the autoimmune disorder. Autoimmune disorders may affect one or multiple organs or tissues, and can result in destruction of body tissues and abnormal organ function and growth. Several autoimmune disorders are discussed elsewhere in this report, including multiple sclerosis, rheumatoid arthritis, and systemic lupus erythematosus. Symptoms of autoimmune disorders can include fatigue, fever, malaise, joint pain, and rashes. Treatments include reduction of symptoms and maintenance of the body's ability to fight disease while controlling the autoimmune process itself.

There is some evidence that cannabinoids may be able to help modulate autoimmune disorders. A study of the effects of cannabis on laboratory rats indicated that, while CBD did not reduce certain immune cells important in fighting against viruses and tumors, it did reduce other cells that are involved in inflammatory, autoimmune, and neurodegenerative diseases.[54] This work has been confirmed in other studies of THC on mouse immune CD4+ cells.[473, 659] In laboratory mice with experimentally induced autoimmune encephalitis, both THC and CBD were able to modulate the immune chemicals that are associated with inflammatory autoimmune diseases.[58, 59]

Additional Autoimmune disorder resources:
American Autoimmune Related Diseases Association: www.aarda.org
National Library of Medicine: www.nlm.nih.gov

Bacterial infections: antibiotic resistant

Bacterial infections are commonly treated with antibiotics, substances that act in various ways to kill or reduce growth of bacterial cells. Unfortunately, because of their rapid generation times, bacteria can evolve resistance to antibiotics and other antimicrobial substances more rapidly than we can develop new treatments against them. Infections caused by resistant microorganisms may not respond to standard treatments, and can cause prolonged illness, and loss of limbs or even death. The World Health Organization indicates that antimicrobial resistance is present in all parts of the world, and is an increasingly serious threat to global public health. One extremely dangerous organism that is becoming resistant to multiple antibiotics is *Mycobacterium tuberculosis*, the bacterium that causes tuberculosis. Another serious and common cause of hospital-acquired infections is methicillin-resistant *Staphylococcus aureus* (MRSA), which is actually resistant to several front-line antibiotics. It can cause skin and other infections, and in hospitals and nursing homes is a cause of bloodstream infections, pneumonia, and infection of surgical wounds. The US CDC indicates that MRSA can be transmitted through direct contact with infected wounds or by sharing personal items that have touched infected skin. Symptoms of MRSA appear initially as a bump or infected area of skin that can be red, swollen, painful, warm, pus-filled, and potentially accompanied by fever. Several cannabinoids are known to have antibacterial properties,[12] and have even proven effective against several MRSA strains.[20]

Additional Antibiotic resistant bacterial infection resources:
US Centers for Disease Control and Prevention: www.cdc.gov
World Health Organization:
www.who.int

Bipolar disorder

Bipolar disorder is also known as manic-depressive disorder. It is a brain disorder that is characterized by severe shifts in mood, activity levels, energy, and ability to carry out daily functions. The National Institute of Mental Health describes symptoms of mania and depression in detail, briefly summarized here:

- *Mania or manic episode*: long period of feeling "high", overly happy or outgoing, extreme irritability, rapid speech, racing thoughts, easily distracted, increased activities, restlessness, decreased sleep, impulsive behaviors, engaging in pleasurable high risk behaviors, having unrealistic belief in one's abilities

- *Depression or depressive episode*: long period of feeling sad or hopeless, loss of interest in normally enjoyable activities, fatigue, difficulty concentrating, remembering, making decisions, changes in eating and sleeping, thoughts of death or suicide, or attempted suicide.

There are different forms of bipolar disorder that have different levels of manic or depressive episodes. Substance abuse is very common among people with bipolar disorder, potentially due to an attempt to self-treat symptoms, but substance abuse can also trigger or prolong bipolar symptoms.

Bipolar disorder is thought to be multifactorial, with genetic tendencies as well as environmental factors involved. Bipolar disorder cannot be cured, and is a lifelong illness, but there can be periods that are symptom free. Various medications are used to help control symptoms, but these can have uncomfortable and occasionally serious side effects. Some types of medications can cause tardive dyskinesia, which manifests as uncontrollable muscle movements. Sometimes side effects are sufficiently severe that patients do not always adhere to treatment regimens. Psychotherapy can also help in combination with medications. A more extreme form of treatment is electroconvulsive therapy (ECT), typically used when other treatments have not been effective. ECT causes some short term side effects such as confusion, disorientation and memory loss.

Case histories of bipolar disorder patients indicate that cannabis can be effective to treat symptoms of mania, depression, or both, and that it may allow for reduced use of medications such as lithium.[686] A comparative study of patients with bipolar disorder and those with schizophrenia found that cannabis was associated with improved neurocognitive function in bipolar disorder, but with decreased function in schizophrenia.[687] Another study of bipolar patients with and without a history of cannabis use disorder indicated that those patients who used cannabis had significantly better attention, cognitive processing speed, and working memory.[688] However, a more recent study of cannabis use and bipolar disorder found that recent cannabis use was significantly associated with lower age at onset of first manic and psychotic episode, but not with onset of first depressive episode. Recent use was also associated with more lifetime suicide attempts.[388] Note that an association does not necessarily mean that cannabis use caused the episodes – an alternative hypothesis could be that of self-medication for individuals with earlier onset or with more suicidal tendencies. Other studies have shown that cannabis use may be associated with higher risk of manic or mixed episodes and/or poorer functioning,[251, 333, 389, 390, 392-394] and there are a few case studies indicating that cannabis use may precipitate bipolar disorder.[391]

Additional Bipolar disorder resources:
American Psychiatric Association:
www.psychiatry.org
Brain & Behavior Research Foundation: bbrfoundation.org
Depression and Bipolar Support Alliance: www.dbsalliance.org
National Institute of Mental Health: www.nimh.nih.gov

Bladder dysfunction

Bladder dysfunction is a term for conditions such as overactive bladder, incontinence, urinary tract obstruction, and neurogenic bladder (when normal nerve or muscle control of bladder is impaired); all of these conditions lead to the bladder being abnormally filled or emptied. Bladder dysfunction can be caused by medications, but is also very common in neurological disorders such as multiple sclerosis (see Multiple Sclerosis, Chapter 3). The effects of cannabis on bladder dysfunction have been of particular use to patients with multiple sclerosis, as it can reduce urinary urgency, incontinence, urinary frequency, and nocturia (being awakened due to need to urinate). A study of the effects of CBD on bladder contractility in rat and human bladder sections that were stimulated with electricity to cause contractions found that CBD was able to significantly reduce contractions.[575] Cannabis-based extracts may be a safe and effective treatment for bladder dysfunction, based on studies of bladder dysfunction in multiple sclerosis patients. Multiple sclerosis patients treated with THC and CBD showed significant improvement in urinary urgency and frequency, number and volume of incontinence episodes, and nocturia, and patients rated pain, spasticity, and quality of sleep as significantly improved. The authors also reported few problematic side effects.[210] In a larger group of 630 multiple sclerosis patients, both oral cannabis extract and THC significantly reduced the urge to urinate relative to a placebo.[581]

Brachial plexus avulsion

The brachial plexus is a bundle of nerves that runs from the upper spine through the neck, and into the armpit and arm. It provides nerve signal conduction from the spine to the shoulder, arm and hand. Brachial plexus avulsion is a severe injury caused when the nerve root is severed from the spinal cord. Motor vehicle accidents are a common cause of brachial plexus avulsion. Without prompt surgical reconnection, brachial plexus avulsion can result in paralysis of the arm, lack of muscle control in hand, wrist or arm, and lack of sensation in arm or hand. Combination therapy with CBD and THC has been shown to reduce spasms and pain in conditions such as brachial plexus avulsion.[207, 500]

Additional Brachial plexus avulsion resources:

National Institute of Neurological Disorder and Stroke: www.ninds.nih.gov

Cerebral malaria

Malaria in humans is caused by infection with the species of the parasite *Plasmodium*. *Plasmodium* species are transmitted by species of *Anopheles* mosquitoes when it takes a blood meal. *Plasmodia* parasites then incubate for a time in the blood of the infected person. Malaria results as the parasite develops in the blood, producing toxic substances that accumulate in the red blood cell; when the parasite multiplies, it breaks the blood cell to release new parasites, also dumping the toxic substances into the blood. The US CDC indicates that malaria can range from uncomplicated, with symptoms of alternating shivering and fever/sweating, fever, headaches, and vomiting, and general fatigue and body aches, to severe, with symptoms including anemia, hypoglycemia, seizures, coma, multiple organ failure, and even death. Although small isolated outbreaks of malaria have occurred in the US, typically the disease is brought in from endemic countries by mosquitoes on an airplane, or by travelers returning from malaria-endemic countries. Malaria is treatable, but drug resistance has become common in the parasites.

Cerebral malaria is a very severe neurological complication of *Plasmodium* infection. More than half a million cases are reported annually, mostly among children in sub-Saharan Africa.[819] The disease causes coma and brain injury, and frequently is fatal. Patients who survive this infection are at risk of neurological and cognitive (thinking) defects, behavioral problems, and epilepsy. A recent study[43] of induced cerebral malaria in mice found that treatment with CBD prevented memory deficits and anxiety behaviors, increased a beneficial protein called brain-derived neurotrophic factor (BDNF, which helps nerve cells grow, mature, and maintain function), and decreased inflammatory chemicals in the brain. The authors found that CBD's neuroprotective effects in the mouse model suggest it to be a useful therapy in this disease.

Additional Cerebral malaria resources:
Bill & Melinda Gates Foundation:
www.gatesfoundation.org
Malaria No More:
www.malarianomore.org
US Centers for Disease Control and Prevention: www.cdc.gov
World Health Organization:
www.who.int

Cerebral Palsy

Cerebral palsy encompasses a group of disorders caused by abnormal brain development or damage to the brain that affects motor control. The US CDC indicates that cerebral palsy is the most common motor disability of childhood. Cerebral palsy can range from mild to severe. Cerebral palsy is characterized by problems with posture and movement, and commonly co-occurs with other related conditions such as intellectual disabilities, seizures, hearing and vision problems, speech problems, and spine and joint problems.

The CDC describes four main types of cerebral palsy, briefly

- Spastic cerebral palsy: most common, affecting about 80% of cerebral palsy patients. Spastic cerebral palsy is characterized by muscle stiffness with resulting movement difficulties. Stiffness can be mainly in the legs, mainly on one side of the body, or in all of the body. People with the type that affects the entire body (spastic quadriplegia) usually cannot walk and typically have intellectual disability, seizures, and vision, hearing, and speech problems.

- Dyskinetic cerebral palsy: characterized by difficulties controlling hand, arm, foot, and leg movements. This results in difficulties sitting and walking, and movements are typically slow and writhing or rapid and jerky. If the face and tongue are affected, the person might have difficulty sucking, swallowing, and talking.

- Ataxic cerebral palsy: characterized by problems with balance and coordination. Symptoms include unsteady gait, and difficulty with quick or controlled movements.

- Mixed cerebral palsy: this is characterized by symptoms of more than one type of cerebral palsy, the most common being a mix of spastic and dyskinetic cerebral palsy.

Cannabis has been found to provide relief from seizures and spasticity in other disorders such as epilepsy, spasticity, and multiple sclerosis (see Chapter 3 for discussion of these conditions). At least one case study showed the benefits of using cannabis in the treatment of co-occurring cerebral palsy and epilepsy.[248] Following oral administration of THC in patients with spasticity conditions, including cerebral palsy, spasms were significantly reduced relative to placebo.[171]

Additional Cerebral palsy resources:
American Academy for Cerebral Palsy and Developmental Medicine:
www.aacpdm.org
Cerebral Palsy Alliance: www.cerebralpalsy.org
CerebralPalsy.org: cerebralpalsy.org
March of Dimes: www.marchofdimes.org
National Institute of Neurological Disorders and Stroke: www.ninds.nih.gov
United Cerebral Palsy: ucp.org
US Centers for Disease Control and Prevention: www.cdc.gov

Chronic Liver Disease (see also Chapter 3 Cirrhosis; Hepatitis C infection)

Chronic liver diseases are caused by viruses (such as hepatitis A, B, or C), medications, toxins, or excess alcohol. They can also be caused by other conditions such as cancer. The US CDC indicates that chronic liver disease and cirrhosis caused some 33,642 deaths in the US in 2011. Chronic liver diseases are discussed in more detail in Chapter 3, Cirrhosis; and Hepatitis C. Studies of hepatitis C in human patients have shown that orally administered cannabinoids can be effective at reducing chemotherapy-induced symptoms of anorexia, nausea and vomiting.[489] A large proportion of hepatitis C virus patients are reported to smoke marijuana to reduce side effects from anti-viral medications , and although at least one study has shown that cannabis may increase severity of hepatitis C disease,[366, 367] other studies have found either no effect of marijuana on disease[548] or survival rates.[691] However, a study of substance abusers found that chronic marijuana use may lead to deleterious liver alterations.[368] In contrast, animal studies of induced chronic liver disease have found that cannabidiol can reverse cognitive and motor effects of the disease,[15] as well as increase the expression levels of brain-derived neurotrophic factor, an important brain protein.[66]

Additional Chronic liver disease resources:
American Liver Foundation: www.liverfoundation.org
Chronic Liver Disease Foundation: www.chronicliverdisease.org
US Centers for Disease Control and Prevention: www.cdc.gov

Chronic Obstructive Pulmonary Disease (COPD)

Chronic obstructive pulmonary disease is also known as COPD, and includes two main conditions: emphysema and chronic bronchitis. In emphysema, the parts of the lungs that hold air (alveoli) become damaged or even destroyed, and this reduces the amount of gas exchange in the lungs. In chronic bronchitis, the lining of the airways (bronchial tubes) become irritated, inflamed, and thickened, with excessive mucus formation. Ultimately, less air flows in and out of the lungs. The National Heart, Lung, and Blood Institute indicates that cigarette smoking is the leading cause of COPD, although long term exposure to pollution, chemical fumes, or dust can also contribute to COPD. People with COPD have difficulty breathing. COPD is the third leading cause of death in the US. There is no cure, and as yet, no way to reverse damage to the airways and lungs. Treatments focus on symptom relief, preventing further damage, and quality of life improvements.

A clinical study of patients with COPD showed that sublingually administered CBD and THC were able to relieve feelings of breathlessness.[692] While smoking anything is contraindicated for COPD patients, a large survey study of marijuana and tobacco smokers found that smoking only marijuana (and not tobacco), was not associated with an increased risk of respiratory symptoms or COPD.[693] Other studies of habitual marijuana smokers have also found no causal role of smoking for COPD,[695] or emphysema, but one did find higher incidence of inflammatory cells, which may lead to lung injury.[694] However, some studies have linked chronic marijuana smoking (for an average of 8.8 years) with lung injury in young people (all younger than 43 years of age),[467] and chronic smokers are more likely to have cough, phlegm, and wheeze.[468] A more recent study of habitual marijuana and tobacco smokers found that current smokers were more likely to have chronic bronchitis, and that cessation of smoking resolved previous symptoms.[466]

Additional Chronic obstructive pulmonary disease resources:
American Lung Association:
www.lung.org
COPD Foundation:
www.copdfoundation.org

National Heart, Lung, and Blood Institute: www.nhlbi.nih.gov
The Global Initiative for Chronic Obstructive Lung Disease:
www.goldcopd.org
US Centers for Disease Control and Prevention: www.cdc.gov
World Health Organization:
www.who.int

Cystic Fibrosis

Cystic fibrosis is a disease of the glands that make mucus and sweat. According to the National Heart, Lung, and Blood Institute, the disease is inherited from parents, and mainly infects the lungs, pancreas, liver, intestines, sinuses, and sex organs. In cystic fibrosis, mucus is much more thick and sticky than normal mucus, and builds up on the lungs and blocks air passages. In addition to blockage of airways, mucus buildup also makes it easy for bacterial infections to take hold, and repeated lung infections can severely damage a patient's lungs over time. Overly thick mucus also blocks the pancreatic ducts, and digestive enzymes cannot reach the intestine, which leads over time to vitamin deficiency and malnutrition because nutrients are not digested properly. Additionally, severe constipation, gas, and swollen, painful belly can result. The sweat glands are also affected in cystic fibrosis, and the person loses large amounts of salt when they sweat, causing problems such as dehydration, increased heart rate, fatigue, weakness, low blood pressure, heat stroke, and even death. People with cystic fibrosis are also at higher risk for diabetes, or osteoporosis and osteopenia (described in Chapter 3, Treatment with AZT, Chemotherapy, Radiotherapy, and Protease Inhibitors).

A study of cannabidiol derivatives on a mouse model showed that intestinal motility (intestinal contractions that propel fecal matter) was inhibited by acting on the peripheral nervous system,[23] and the authors suggest that complex disorders such as inflammatory bowel disease and cystic fibrosis may benefit from development of cannabis-based medicines. However, smoked marijuana may be contraindicated for cystic fibrosis due to potential lung damage from inhaled smoke. A case study of a 23 year old man reports that he developed lung damage (termed "bong lung") from repeated smoking of cannabis.[470]

Additional Cystic fibrosis resources:
American Lung Association:
www.lung.org
Cystic Fibrosis Foundation: www.cff.org
Cystic Fibrosis.com:
www.cysticfibrosis.com
March of Dimes:
www.marchofdimes.org
National Heart, Lung, and Blood Institute: www.nhlbi.nih.gov

Degenerative disc disease

Degeneration of the discs between the vertebral bones of the spine is a natural part of aging, but in some individuals the process may be painful, and may be accompanied by osteoarthritis. According to Spine-Health, the pain associated with disc degeneration is thought to arise from inflammation and instability due to the wearing down of the disc. In addition, there may also be muscle spasms as the body attempts to stabilize the spine, and these can be painful. Treatment is typically medications to control inflammation and pain, exercise and physical therapy, and in severe cases, surgery.

The anti-inflammatory, anti-spasmodic, and analgesic properties of cannabis that are discussed elsewhere (see Tables 1 and 2 and sections in Chapter 3 on Arthritis; Muscle Spasms; Pain: chronic/severe/intractable) make it useful for treatment of degenerative disc disease. Additionally, a study of laboratory rats with induced disc injury found that injection of cannabidiol significantly reduced the effects of the injury.[698]

Additional Degenerative disc disease resources:
Spine-Health: www.spine-health.com

Depression

Depression is a serious mental illness that interferes with daily life. The National Institute of Mental Health describes the symptoms of depression, and discusses several forms of depressive disorders, briefly described here. Symptoms of depression are of a persistent nature, and include sad, anxious, empty, hopeless, guilty, worthless, or helpless feelings, irritability and restlessness, loss of interest in once pleasurable activities, fatigue, difficulty concentrating, insomnia or excessive sleeping, overeating or loss of appetite loss, and thoughts of suicide or suicide attempts. Types of depression include

- *Major depression*: can occur in one or more episodes throughout life. Severe symptoms that interfere with daily functionality.

- *Persistent depressive disorder*: symptoms that last for at least 2 years, and may include periods of major depression.

- *Psychotic depression*: depression along with some form of psychosis such as disturbing false beliefs, break with reality, or hallucinations.

- *Postpartum depression*: overwhelming symptoms of depression brought along by hormonal and physical changes of giving birth, as well as the responsibility of caring for a newborn.

- *Seasonal affective disorder* (SAD): depression symptoms during winter months, due to reduced sunlight.

- *Bipolar disorder*: includes depression as well as extreme highs (see Bipolar Disorder).

Depression is thought to be caused by genetic, biological, environmental, and psychological factors. Brain scans show that people with depression have differences in their mood, cognitive, sleep, appetite, and behavior controlling portions of the brain. The National Institute of Mental Health indicates that major depressive disorder affects about 6.7% of adults each year, and women are more likely than men to experience depression during their lifetime. Among adolescents, 3.3% are estimated to have experienced a serious depressive disorder.

Treatments for depression include psychotherapy and medications, some of which have serious side effects and which cause serious withdrawal effects if discontinued. In cases of extreme depression that is unresponsive to psychotherapy and medication, brain stimulation techniques such as electroconvulsive therapy may be effective.

Analyses of various populations with depression indicate that cannabis is used as a coping mechanism for depression and/or stress.[701, 707] A survey of nearly 3000 United Kingdom medical cannabis users found that depression is a common condition for which patients seek medicinal cannabis.[700] In a study of depression and veterans, individuals who expected positive results from using cannabis used more cannabis to self-medicate their depression.[699] At least two studies in animal models have confirmed that cannabinoids have antidepressant-like effects, and can contribute to mood elevation.[99, 117] However, a study of adolescent rats found that chronic THC administration caused "behavioral despair" among females (but not males).[349]

While there have been some indications that cannabis use, particularly in adolescence, may precipitate depressive symptoms or even suicidal ideation,[350, 354, 356] multiple studies have found that cannabis use in and of itself does not increase depressive and/or suicidal tendencies,[703, 705, 706, 708-712] and in fact, young people using cannabis may be attempting to self-medicate for pre-existing depression.[704] Further, the association between adolescent cannabis use and later major depression is at least partially explained by what is termed "psychosocial failure" (dropping out of school, persistent unemployment, or engagement in criminal activities.)[353] A survey of over 173,000 individuals in the US did find a modest increased risk of depression in adulthood among individuals who had smoked cannabis as adolescents,[351] but it is not at all clear that there is any causal relationship. In cases in which adolescent cannabis use does seem to precipitate depression, a molecular biological study found that a specific genetic variation may underlie this phenomenon[352]—in other words, people with a certain genetic makeup may be more prone to depression that cannabis use can initiate. In another attempt to understand a functional relationship between marijuana use and depression, a study of marijuana use changes aspects of the brain in young people with major depressive disorder.[355]

Several studies of patients with disorders such as bipolar, schizophrenia, and depression consistently find that, while cannabis use may predict an increase in psychosis symptoms, it does not increase symptoms of depression.[410, 411, 702]

Additional Depression resources:
American Psychiatric Association:
www.psychiatry.org
Brain & Behavior Research Foundation: bbrfoundation.org
Depression and Bipolar Support Alliance: www.dbsalliance.org
National Institute of Mental Health: www.nimh.nih.gov

Diabetes

Diabetes is a disease in which sugar builds up in the blood instead of being sent to the cells for energy. Blood glucose (sugar) levels increase to unhealthy levels when the body either does not make enough insulin, which helps process glucose into energy, or when the body cannot properly use the insulin that it makes. The organ that makes insulin is called the pancreas. Cells that do not get energy cannot function properly, and that means that the organs cannot function properly. Diabetes is thus a serious disease that can lead to heart disease, blindness, kidney failure, amputations, and painful peripheral neuropathy (see Chapter 3, Peripheral Neuropathy). The US CDC reports that diabetes is the seventh leading cause of death in the United States.

The National Diabetes Information Clearinghouse at the National Institutes of Health describes three main types of diabetes. These are briefly discussed here:

- *Type 1 Diabetes* is also known as "juvenile diabetes", although it can develop in adults as well. In type 1 diabetes, the body's own immune system mistakenly attacks and destroys the cells that make insulin.

- *Type 2 diabetes* usually develops following insulin resistance. Insulin resistance means that the body is not properly using insulin to convert glucose into energy, resulting in an increased need for insulin to get glucose into cells. The pancreas makes more and more insulin to try and keep up with the demand, but ultimately it cannot make enough.

People of any age can get type 2 diabetes, but it is more common in middle aged and older people, as well as in overweight and inactive people. Other potential causes of insulin resistance are certain diseases, use of steroids, use of certain medications, sleep apnea, and tobacco smoking.

- *Gestational diabetes* can occur during pregnancy due to hormones that lead to insulin resistance. If the pancreas cannot make sufficient insulin during pregnancy, gestational diabetes will develop. Although gestational diabetes usually goes away after the baby is born, the mother is more likely to develop type 2 diabetes eventually, and any of her babies are also more likely to develop obesity and type 2 diabetes later in life. Women who gain too much weight during pregnancy, or who are already overweight or obese have a higher chance of gestational diabetes.

Treatments for diabetes involve insulin injections for type 1 diabetes, and for all types, medications, healthy food choices, physical activity, controlling blood pressure, and controlling cholesterol. Cannabis use has been associated with a lower prevalence of diabetes mellitus.[713] A large study of over 4500 current or past cannabis users found that current users had 16% lower fasting insulin levels and smaller waist circumference.[312] Cannabis use in an Inuit population from Nunavik was associated with lower BMI, lower percent fat mass, lower fasting insulin, and lower insulin resistance.[311] Research in mouse models of diabetes has found that cannabidiol can reduce insulitis (inflammation of certain pancreas regions that produce insulin) and inhibited the inflammatory response, resulting in a decreased incidence of diabetes,[97] and reduced heart problems associated with diabetes.[81] A study in lean and obese rats also found that THC and CBN can reduce blood clots, which are a concern in type 2 diabetes.[113] A laboratory study of mouse adipocyte (fat) cells showed that those exposed to THC extract delayed adipogenesis (development of fat cells) and improved the ability of the adipocytes to respond to insulin stimulation.[714] A single study of cannabis-based extract on 30 subjects with painful diabetic peripheral neuropathy found that it was no more effective than placebo, but the authors caution that the study was confounded by depression,[237] and this is important to take in consideration along with the fact that many studies have found cannabis to be beneficial in peripheral neuropathic pain (see Chapter 3, Peripheral Neuropathy).

Additional Diabetes resources:
American Diabetes Association:
www.diabetes.org
American Heart Association:
www.heart.org
International Diabetes Federation: www.idf.org
National Diabetes Information Clearinghouse: diabetes.niddk.nih.gov
Us Centers for Disease Control and Prevention: www.cdc.gov
World Health Organization:
www.who.int

Diarrhea

The World Health Organization defines diarrhea as the passage of 3 or more loose or liquid stools per day, or more frequently than is normal for that person. Diarrheas can be accompanied by cramping, bloating, and nausea. Diarrheas are often symptoms of gastrointestinal infections from bacteria, viruses, and parasites. When diarrhea is severe, it can lead to dehydration and can be life-threatening in children, malnourished people, and those with impaired immunity. Certain other conditions and medications can cause diarrheas, and in Chapter 3, we discussed the efficacy of cannabis for treating various gastrointestinal disorders and symptoms (see Crohn's disease; Inflammatory bowel disease; Nausea; Vomiting). In a laboratory rat study, an extract of medicinal cannabis administered into the colon was able to improve diarrhea, weight loss, and healing of ulcerated tissues. It was also able to prevent gastric distention-induced pain via the CB2 receptors.[252] Two other studies showed that inhaled cannabis may contribute to diarrhea, however. In a study in which dogs were made to inhale four marijuana cigarettes per day for 9 months, food consumption at first increased and was accompanied by diarrhea, but then decreased.[820] Another study in a vaccine development program found that heavy use of cannabis was associated with more voluminous diarrhea, but only after infection with the bacterium *Vibrio cholera* (which causes cholera) or enterotoxigenic *Escherichia coli* bacteria (which on their own cause voluminous diarrhea).[715]

Additional Diarrhea resources:
World Health Organization:
www.who.int

Herpes virus infection

Herpes viruses comprise a large group of viruses that are found in many animal species, including humans. They are highly adapted to their hosts, and an animal species cannot be successfully infected with the herpes virus adapted to another species. Most herpes viruses infect the cells throughout an organism's body, have elaborate ways to modulate the host's responses to the infection, and can thus establish a lifelong latent (not always active) infection that can subsequently reactivate.[821] There are eight types of herpesviruses that infect humans: herpes simplex virus type 1, herpes simplex virus type 2, varicella-zoster virus, Epstein-Barr virus (causes infectious mononucleosis), cytomegalovirus, human herpesvirus 6, human herpesvirus 7, and human herpesvirus 8 (also known as Kaposi sarcoma-associated herpesvirus). Herpes viruses typically require intimate contact, with the exception of varicella-zoster virus (that which causes chicken pox and shingles), which can be spread through aerosols (coughs, sneezing, etc.). Extensive information about these viruses can be found in the book *Human Herpesviruses: Biology, Therapy, and Immunoprophylaxis* edited by A. Arvin and others, and available through the National Library of Medicine at www.ncbi.nlm.nih.gov/books/NBK47406/#c01bny-j8s-dd3-fg6. A brief description of herpesvirus infections is distilled from this volume here:

- *Herpes simplex virus (types 1 and 2) infections*: both of these viruses commonly cause oral or genital infection, and are transmitted from close contact with an infected person. They can also cause infection of the eye, the central nervous system. The infection is commonly mild but can be severe, especially in patients with HIV infections.

- *Varicella-zoster virus*: chickenpox is typically a childhood disease that can resolve itself unless it is severe; infection with varicella-zoster virus can be serious in adults and in immune compromised children. Chickenpox is characterized by a rash that is quite uncomfortable. After the disease resolves, the virus goes latent and may later reactivate, causing herpes zoster, or "shingles". Shingles is common in elderly and HIV-infected people. The skin and other areas of the body become inflamed and can be very painful.

- *Epstein-Barr virus*: infection with Epstein-Barr virus causes infectious mononucleosis and is very common in humans. In healthy individuals it may cause no or minimal symptoms and usually resolves on its own. Infectious mononucleosis is characterized by fever, fatigue, sore throat, and sore lymph nodes. There can be complications of severe disease that include neurological complications such as peripheral neuropathy, blood conditions, rupture of the spleen, and respiratory and liver complications.

- *Cytomegalovirus*: cytomegalovirus is transmitted through blood or bodily fluids, and the infection can cause a disease that is similar to infectious mononucleosis and that has a range of severity. It can be particularly serious in HIV-infected and immunocompromised patients. It can also be passed on to a fetus and either cause no problems, or cause abortion, stillbirth, or death after birth. In healthy people, the infection may have no symptoms or only minimal symptoms, but in immunocompromised cytomegalovirus can affect the lungs, gastrointestinal tract, or central nervous system, and may be fatal.

- *Human herpesviruses 6 and 7*: these are common in children, and typically cause ear infections, fevers, or a rash known as roseola. Human herpesvirus 6 infection can rarely be serious, and may cause encephalitis or seizures.

Human herpesvirus 8: this virus is transmitted through bodily fluids or among injection drug users, and rarely causes illness in immune competent individuals. In AIDS patients, however, human herpesvirus 8 causes Kaposi Sarcoma and other lymphomas. Kaposi Sarcoma is a type of cancer that has skin lesions, especially on the face and trunk, and may also infect the lymph nodes and gastrointestinal tract.

Many of the herpes viruses cause minimal symptoms that can resolve themselves in immune competent individuals, and treatment often focuses on relief of symptoms. In severe cases, antiviral medications can be used to prevent viral replication and spread.

Cannabis may be effective at preventing at least some types of herpes virus infections. In cultured tissues that were infected with gamma herpesviruses, THC inhibited the replication of the viruses, while not affecting the growth of the host cells themselves.(163) However, early studies in mice found that THC suppressed the immune system sufficiently to render the mice more susceptible to herpes simplex virus type 2.[374] Other studies of mice infected with herpes simplex virus type 1 found that THC prevented certain immune cells from killing the infected cells.[371, 372] Further, mice co-infected with an immune depressive virus (Friend leukemia virus) and herpes simplex virus were treated with THC, which decreased certain mouse immune cells and allowed the two viruses to induce more rapid mortality; the authors of this study suggest that in humans with HIV infection, THC could act similarly in conjunction with opportunistic infectious agents to aid the progression of the infection to overt AIDS.[373]

Additional Herpes virus resources:
American Academy of Dermatology: www.aad.org
United States Centers for Disease Control and Prevention: www.cdc.gov

Hiccups: Intractable

Persistent hiccups may be associated with an underlying problem or certain medications, and intractable hiccups are a rare complication of AIDS.[822] There is a single case report of an AIDS patient who developed hiccups that lasted for 8 days; this patient had never previously smoked marijuana, and after smoking some, hiccups ceased.[717] The hiccups recurred on two successive days, he smoked marijuana each day and the hiccupping stopped, and on the second day, the hiccups did not return.

Hypertension

Hypertension is more commonly known as high blood pressure, a condition that the US CDC reports is common in about 1 out of every 3 US adults. High blood pressure increases risk for heart disease and stroke, and it is more common in older people and in people with a family history of hypertension. People with diabetes mellitus are at increased risk for hypertension, as are people who are obese, physically inactive, use tobacco, drink excessively, and those who regularly consume foods high in sodium and low in potassium. Lifestyle changes and medications can be very effective at treating hypertension.

There is some evidence that cannabis may help to control blood pressure. In hypertensive laboratory rats, THC at a moderate dose was able to significantly lower the average blood pressure.[121, 189] Hemp seed meal protein hydrolysate fed to young hypertensive rats significantly reduced blood pressure compared to rats eating a normal diet.[264] In a study of 13 daily cannabis users, blood pressure was found to significantly increase during cannabis abstinence.[718] In human hypertensive subjects with glaucoma, smoked cannabis lowers both intraocular pressure and blood pressure[265, 266] (See Chapter 3, Glaucoma, for more information). However, in individuals who smoke both tobacco and cannabis, hypertension has been reported,[720] and intravenously administered THC was associated with development of hypertension in one study.[370]

Additional Hypertension resources:
American Heart Association:
www.heart.org
American Society of Hypertension: www.ash-us.org
US Centers for Disease Control and Prevention: www.cdc.gov

Night Vision

Vision at night may be impaired in certain conditions such as retinitis pigmentosa, diabetes, or cataracts.

Smoked cannabis and oral THC have both been found to improve night vision in humans, possibly in a dose-dependent manner (more cannabis/THC leads to better vision).[193, 721]

Nystagmus

Nystagmus is a condition in which the eyes make involuntary repetitive eye movements, resulting in problems with visual acuity and depth perception. The American Optometric Association indicates that nystagmus usually develops in childhood (known as congenital nystagmus or spasmus nutans), or can be acquired either in adulthood or childhood (known as acquired nystagmus). Nystagmus is caused by problems with the visual pathway from the eye to the brain, lack of development of normal eye movement control, central nervous system diseases, congenital cataracts, albinism, multiple sclerosis, stroke, inner ear inflammation, and medications such as anti-epilepsy drugs. There is no cure for nystagmus, although surgery, eyeglasses and contact lenses can help improve associated vision conditions.

Cannabis may be beneficial in some cases of nystagmus. Case studies have found that smoked cannabis reduced nystagmus in a multiple sclerosis patient,[589] and in a young man with congenital nystagmus.[722] However, another case of gaze-evoked nystagma was reported in an adult male who developed the visual disturbances after marijuana use,[395] although it is uncertain that there was a causal association.

Additional Nystagmus resources:
American Association for Pediatric Opthalmology and Strabismus: www.aapos.org
American Optometric Association: www.aoa.org

Obesity

Obesity is a term used for a range of weight for a given height that is not considered healthy. Obesity is typically measured for adults by using the body mass index (BMI), which for the most part correlates with amount of body fat. A normal BMI for an adult is between 18.5 and 24.9; below that is underweight, above that is overweight. If the BMI is 30 or greater, the person is considered obese. (Certain categories of people, such as athletes, may have BMIs that differ from the standard chart due to their higher proportions of muscle tissue). The US CDC reports that in 2009-2010, more than one-third of adults and 17% of children and adolescents in the United States were obese. Abdominal fat is also important to consider when assessing obesity, because it is associated with certain diseases.

Obesity is associated with serious health consequences. The CDC lists the following conditions that have increased risk among obese people: coronary heart disease and stroke, Type 2 diabetes, certain cancers, hypertension, dyslipidemia (abnormal amounts of fat in the blood), liver and gallbladder disease, sleep apnea and respiratory problems, osteoarthritis, and gynecological problems. There can be many causes for obesity, but essentially an energy imbalance is at the core of the issue-more energy is taken in than put out in daily activities. There can be some genetic, disease, and medication issues as well that contribute to obesity.

Although it might seem counterintuitive, given that cannabis smoking is orexigenic and has a reputation for causing "the munchies", a recent study pointed out that the prevalence of obesity is actually much lower in cannabis users than non-cannabis users,[309] a difference that could not be accounted for by tobacco smoking status, age, or sex.[308] The authors suggest that THC or a THC/CBD combination may produce weight loss and prove a useful therapeutic for the treatment of obesity. A large sample of female humans receiving treatment for weight management found that lower body mass index was associated with higher marijuana use; the more obese women were significantly less likely to have used marijuana in the past year.[313] Cannabis use has also been associated with decreased probability of obesity in a large sample of African American and Puerto Rican young adults.[723] Treatment with THCV of twenty healthy adult volunteers was able to increase responses to aversive stimuli (and thus make the people not want to eat a pleasant food like chocolate).[192] A survey of over 5000 young people, however, found that cannabis use from ages 12 to 18 was associated with increased risk of obesity in young adulthood (ages 20 to 24).[314] A study of 72 adults assessed metabolism and chronic cannabis smoking, and found that smokers had higher levels of visceral adiposity (fat in the abdomen) and fat tissue insulin resistance, but they did not have higher levels of liver problems, pancreatic function, insulin insensitivity or glucose intolerance relative to controls.[315]

In laboratory studies, cannabinoids have been shown to reduce weight in animals. Pure THCV reduced appetite and weight in laboratory mice, although THCV-rich cannabis extract did not have this effect, suspected by the authors to be due to THC also in the extract – when they administered CBD as well, appetite suppression and weight loss continued. This effect is thought to have been due to the effects of the cannabinoids on the CB1 receptors.[724] In a study of obese laboratory rats, cannabis extract injections changed the gene expression in treated rats relative to control rats, and slowed weight gain and protected cells of the pancreas that are involved in insulin release from negative effects of obesity.[310]

Additional Obesity resources:
American Heart Association:
www.heart.org
American Psychological Association: www.apa.org
Obesity Action Coalition:
www.obesityaction.org
The Obesity Society: www.obesity.org
US Centers for Disease Control and Prevention: www.cdc.gov
World Health Organization:
www.who.int
World Obesity Federation:
www.worldobesity.org

Opioid dependence

Opioids (and opiates, which are derived from the poppy plant) are substances that attach to receptors in the brain, spinal cord, gastrointestinal tract, and other organs, and they affect areas of the brain that receive pain signals and that regulate emotion. Opioids are often used to treat pain, and some of them can also help relieve severe coughs and diarrhea. Commonly known opiates are morphine, heroin, and codeine. Commonly known opioids are hydrocodone and oxycodone. These drugs can be very effective analgesics, but large doses can impair breathing and cause death. Long term use of opioids can also affect the amount of oxygen that reaches the brain and cause brain damage, neurological problems, and coma. Long term use may also cause deterioration of parts of the brain, which affects ability to make decisions, regulate behavior, and appropriately respond to stressful situations. Because opioids can also affect brain regions that are involved in reward feelings, people can feel euphoric after taking them, and the drugs have a high possibility for addiction or dependence. The National Institute on Drug Abuse describes the difference between addiction and dependence: physical dependence occurs when the body makes normal adaptations to a drug after chronic exposure – it is accompanied by a need to take higher doses of the drug over time to achieve the same effect, and if the drug is abruptly reduced or stopped, withdrawal symptoms can occur. Addiction can include physical dependence, but is different in that it is characterized by compulsive drug seeking and use even in the face of serious consequences. It can be incredibly difficult for someone with physical dependence to cease using an opioid. Common withdrawal symptoms from opioids include restlessness, pain in muscles and bones, insomnia, diarrhea, nausea and vomiting, cold flashes with goose bumps, and involuntary leg movements.

Treatments for addiction to opioids include psychotherapy and certain medications. Naltrexone is one medication that is used to prevent the opioid from activating the receptors. Methadone is used to eliminate withdrawal symptoms and reduce drug cravings because it acts on the same targets in the brain as the other opioids do. None of these treatments has perfect efficacy, however, and patients may have trouble tolerating or adhering to treatment regimens.

There have been some concerns that exposure to cannabis, especially THC, might increase addiction to opioids, but studies in animal models have found either no such effect,[727] or even that THC might be beneficial in treatment of opioid dependence. An early study on an induced morphine withdrawal mouse model showed that THC reduced withdrawal behaviors.[199] Administration of THC to morphine-addicted laboratory rats was able to reduce withdrawal symptoms,[148-150] and addition of CBD or CBN additionally decreased symptoms, although CBN and CBD had different effects.[725] Another study of heroin self-administration in laboratory rats demonstrated that CBD reduced heroin-seeking behavior, even after 2 weeks of administration. Neurobiological alterations were also associated with the CBD effects on behavior, and the authors suggest that CBD may be prove useful to treat heroin craving and relapse.

In humans though, study results have been mixed. A 1998 report found that cannabis users were at greater risk of relapse to heroin use.[398] Other studies of human detoxification patients found that intermittent cannabis users were significantly more likely to remain on their treatment programs for opioid dependence.[202, 683] However, cannabis use after discharge from inpatient treatment for cocaine, alcohol, and/or heroin dependence was associated with relapse of alcohol and cocaine use, but not heroin,[396] and in a survey study of 89 opioid dependent outpatients, 37.5% self-reported that cannabis use worsened their withdrawal symptoms.[397] Other studies in humans have found no association between cannabis use and opioid craving/withdrawal,[726] or that cannabis use in and of itself does not associate with negative opioid detoxification outcomes.[533, 728-730]

Additional Opioid dependence resources:
National Institute on Drug Abuse: www.drugabuse.gov
World Health Organization:
www.who.int

Pain: acute

Acute pain is that which begins suddenly, is usually sharp, and tends to be caused by an event such as a burn, cut, broken bone, surgery, or dental work. Acute pain resolves when its underlying cause is removed or has healed. In Chapter 3 we discussed the uses of cannabis for chronic pain, but there is some evidence that cannabinoids may be useful for treatment of acute pain as well. Smoking of cannabis and its effects on pain perception was examined in five regular cannabis users, and cannabis produced significant dose-dependent antinociception (more cannabis gave less pain perception).[145] A study of 65 surgery patients found that there was a dose-related improvement in pain relief (higher doses gave more relief) and pain intensity, and that the doses were equivalent to many routinely used pain medications without frequent adverse effects.[223] A controlled human trial of 15 volunteers found that smoked cannabis significantly reduced experimentally-induced pain after 45 minutes; there was a dose effect of cannabis, with no effect at a low amount of cannabis, decreased pain at a moderate dose, and high doses actually increasing pain.[619] Other studies have found no pain relief properties from cannabis[732] or THC extract,[731] and an early study of 16 habitual cannabis smokers found that moderate levels of cannabis may enhance pain perception.[369]

Prostatitis: chronic

Chronic prostatitis is also known as pelvic pain syndrome, and involves the prostate gland and/or other parts of the male lower urinary tract or genitals. It is not the same as bacterial prostatitis (which is caused by an infection with bacteria). Chronic prostatitis can be caused by previous bacterial prostatitis infections, irritation of the genital or urinary area from by various means, parasites, viruses, or problems with the pelvic floor muscles. The National Library of Medicine indicates that life stresses and emotional factors may also be involved in chronic prostatitis. Symptoms include blood in semen and/or urine, painful bowel movements, painful ejaculation, genital and lower back pain, and urination problems. Chronic prostatitis is reportedly difficult to cure, so treatment focuses on medications for symptom relief. In rare cases in older men, surgery may be performed. A survey of almost 350 men with chronic prostatitis or pelvic pain syndrome indicated that nearly half used cannabis to help with their moods, sleep, pain, and muscle spasms, and of the cannabis users, more than half found it somewhat/very effective for symptom improvement.[618]

Additional Chronic prostatitis resources:
National Library of Medicine:
www.nlm.nih.gov
Prostatitis Foundation: prostatitis.org
Prostatitis Network:
www.chronicprostatitis.com

Psoriasis

Psoriasis is an autoimmune disorder that affects the skin (see also Autoimmune Disorders). It speeds up the growth cycle of skin cells, and causes red, raised, scaly patches. Severity ranges from mild to severe. It may feel like itching, burning, or stinging. The US CDC reports that about 10-20% of people with psoriasis will also have psoriatic arthritis, which is a type of arthritis different from osteoarthritis and rheumatoid arthritis. (Psoriatic arthritis can range from mild to severe, and causes swelling, stiffness, tenderness, and reduced mobility of affected joints.) Treatments for mild psoriasis focus upon topically applied special creams, ointments, and shampoos to control the patches. For moderate or severe psoriasis, light therapy and prescription drugs that affect the entire body. A study on human skin cell lines found that cannabinoids THC, CBD, CBN, and CBG all helped to reduce proliferation of the cells that contribute to psoriasis.[733]

Additional Psoriasis resources:
American Academy of Dermatology: www.aad.org
National Institute of Arthritis and Musculoskeletal and Skin Diseases: www.niams.nih.gov
National Psoriasis Foundation: www.psoriasis.org
US Centers for Disease Control and Prevention: www.cdc.gov

Schizophrenia

Schizophrenia is a disabling brain disorder that is characterized by altered thinking, language, emotional, perception and behavior disruptions, and an altered sense of self. It typically includes psychotic episodes of hallucinations or delusions. Psychotic episodes can be distressing and even terrifying. The World Health Organization indicates that more than 21 million people in the world are affected by schizophrenia, and although it is treatable, half of the people living with the condition do not receive care for it. The National Institute of Mental Health estimates that some 1% of people in the US are afflicted with schizophrenia. The disease makes it very difficult for someone to conduct everyday life, care for oneself, and hold a job. Schizophrenia is thought to be caused by an interaction between genetic predisposition and environmental factors such as early exposure to some infections, malnutrition early in life, including in utero, problems during childbirth, and psychological trauma and stress. The National Institute of Mental Health reports that characteristics of brains of people with schizophrenic are altered relative to those without the disorder – chemical reactions seem to be imbalanced, some areas of the brain are larger, some have less dense gray matter (involved in signal processing), and some areas have altered levels of activity. These changes are thought to occur during brain development before birth, and changes that occur during puberty may trigger symptoms of schizophrenia.

Schizophrenia symptoms are divided into three broad categories, discussed in detail on the National Institute of Mental Health website, and briefly described here.

- *Positive symptoms* are psychotic behaviors that can cause the person to be disconnected from reality.
  - *Hallucinations* are sensory perceptions of things that are not there. Most common is hearing voices, but there are also visual, smell, and touch hallucinations as well.
  - *Delusions* are strong convictions in something that is against commonly accepted reality or rationality, such as believing other people are reading one's mind, or that one is a historical person. People may have paranoid delusions, in which they think that someone is trying to harm them in some way.
  - *Thought disorders* occur when someone has unusual or dysfunctional ways of thinking, such as an inability to organize thoughts, or to continue with a thought, or making up meaningless words.
  - *Movement disorders* are unusual or inappropriate body movements, such as extreme repetition of certain motions, or catatonia (the person does not move or respond to others).

- *Negative symptoms* are disrupted emotions and behaviors such as flat affect (no facial movement or talking monotonously), lack of pleasure, lack of ability to plan and sustain activities, and speaking little. Negative symptoms make everyday tasks difficult or impossible.

- *Cognitive symptoms* include difficulty understanding information and making decisions with it, difficulty focusing or paying attention, and difficulty remembering and using information immediately after learning it.

Schizophrenia is treated with antipsychotic medications and psychosocial interventions to help with everyday life. There are quite a few antipsychotic medications, but not everyone responds to them, and they can have significant side effects. A serious side effect of clozapine, for example, is agranulocytosis, which is a loss of immune cells. Other side effects include drowsiness, dizziness, blurred vision, rapid heartbeat, sun sensitivity, skin rashes, menstrual problems, weight gain, rigidity, muscle spasms and tremors, restlessness and tardive dyskinesia (uncontrollable muscle movements).

About a third of schizophrenia patients' symptoms are not sufficiently controlled with standard antipsychotic medications.[84] Research results on the effects of cannabis on schizophrenia have been mixed. Schizophrenia patients who use cannabis report that it benefits clarity of voices, control of symptoms, promotes feeling normal, improves cognitive function, increases energy, and reduces psychological pain.[750] A meta-analysis confirmed that patients experience fewer symptoms,[752] although in other studies cannabis has been associated with certain motor impairments in schizophrenic patients,[378] and schizophrenia inpatients in one study reported that cannabis use exacerbated their symptoms.[458] Cannabis use has been identified as a risk factor for schizophrenia in numerous studies[413, 414, 421, 428, 804, 805] and may bring forward age of onset of schizophrenia, [386, 426, 429, 435, 436, 444, 448, 453, 792, 793] especially if certain other illicit drugs are also used.[432, 438] Other studies have found that chronic cannabis use is associated with paranoia, psychotic and/or schizotypal symptoms or traits,[317, 333, 384, 385, 410, 412, 416, 420, 422, 423, 430, 434, 462, 798, 806] particularly in young people. [409, 411, 417, 419, 437, 439, 440, 442, 443, 447, 451, 783] A large study of prenatal cannabis exposure found the exposure to be significantly associated with risk of developing psychotic symptoms.[463] The follow-up risk of cannabis use associated psychosis converting into schizophrenia was measured at 46% in a large study of discharged hospital patients.[431] Use of cannabis has also been associated with relapse of psychotic symptoms following treatment,[418, 457,]

[459, 789] and with more severe course and prognosis of schizophrenia. [425, 446, 449, 452, 807]

It is important to note that although individuals who use cannabis are more likely to develop schizophrenia, in and of itself, cannabis use is not thought to cause psychosis (although see [459, 460, 461] for an alternate view), but rather is thought to be one of many interacting factors that lead to the condition. [441, 445, 450, 454, 455, 672, 734] A recent large sample of adult cannabis users found that cannabis use was not associated with psychosis unless alcohol was also used.[782] One explanation for the differing associations between cannabis and psychosis may be that certain genetic variants interact with cannabis use in the adolescent brain to increase schizophrenia susceptibility.[379, 762, 808] A study of the CB1 receptor variants in schizophrenia patients found that heavy cannabis use among persons that have certain genetic variations may contribute to brain white matter deficits and cognitive impairment. Changes in CB1 receptor density in areas the brain have been noted in areas of the brain associated with schizophrenia, and in cannabis users.[803] A matched sibling case-control study found no evidence for a genotype-environment relationship though, while cannabis use was associated with schizophrenia.[800] The correlation between schizophrenia and cannabis may, however, be due to similar genetic predispositions for both, rather than a causal association.[761] Brain chemicals important for growth and maintenance of neurons (and thus for signaling) are also found to be adversely affected in cannabis smokers.[386, 801] Another study hypothesizes that exposure to exocannabinoids (such as from cannabis) during adolescence could adversely affect the immune system and lead to a vulnerability to psychosis.[784]

Laboratory animal research has shown that CBD relieves anxiety and emotional processing impairment in models of schizophrenia,[62, 65] potentially by reducing sensorimotor gating deficits (sensory gating filters out overloading information in the brain).[47, 747] (A study in humans also found that sensory gating was different in heavy cannabis and non-cannabis users, regardless of schizophrenia status.)[382] A study in which the relationship of schizophrenia and inflammation of glial cells found that CBD was able to attenuate induced changes in the glial cells, and to reduce behavioral and expression disruptions.[48] In mice, chronic adolescent exposure to cannabinoids permanently altered neural activity in the prefrontal cortex of the adult brain. The same alterations were not found when the cannabinoid exposure was during adulthood.[786] To examine the relationship between adolescent cannabis use and later schizophrenia, treatment of adolescent rats with THC was found to alter adolescent behavior, and reduce neuronal transmission in the part of the adult brain related to schizophrenia.[785]

Early studies of schizophrenic patients found that those who used substances, including cannabis, had overall better prognoses and less severe characteristics of schizophrenia.[738, 739, 755] In a study of African schizophrenia patients, cannabis use had an apparent protective effect against involuntary movements.[748] Research on patients with a first episode of psychotic illness shows that current or recent cannabis use was associated with clinical features that may have a better outcome,[736, 749, 754] and several studies on patients and controls found that among the schizophrenia patients, those who use cannabis have enhanced cognitive functioning[737, 742-746, 751, 753, 756] (although some studies find lower cognitive functioning,424, 687 especially with current users)[347] – the relationship between cannabis use, schizophrenia, and neurocognitive function is thought to be predicted by illness-related traits that are present early in life.[433] A study of over 74 cannabis users and controls found that the increase in cognitive functioning is associated with fewer gray matter deficits in schizophrenia patients who use cannabis.[741] However, neuroimaging studies have found that semantic memory is impaired while using cannabis, but when not intoxicated, this effect disappeared.[797] Cannabis exposure is associated with areas of lower brain grey matter, [377, 383, 387, 788, 790, 796, 823] and with altered chemical activity in parts of the brain, [296, 380, 802]although CBD had neuroprotective effects in another part of the brain.[296] Schizophrenia itself is associated with high levels of a protein called CCL11 in the blood, and a study of 87 volunteers found that current cannabis users had significantly higher levels of blood CCL11.[787]

A study of 762 patients with psychotic disorders found that cannabis users had a significantly lower risk of mortality compared to non-users who had similar symptoms and treatments.[740] Studies of humans in which cannabinoids have been analyzed individually show that THC may be the cause of anxiety, acute psychosis, and other schizophrenia symptoms, [322, 381, 799, 824] and intravenously administered THC in healthy individuals has been associated with schizophrenia-like symptoms,[415, 795] and with para-noia in patients with paranoid ideation.[323] Cannabidiol, on the other hand, may help to attenuate or even protect from psychosis.[55, 74, 75, 101] A study of 48 volunteers with schizotypy were administered THC, CBD, or THC+CBD and their ability to process the emotional affect of others was measured – THC alone was detrimental to facial recognition, while CBD improved it, and THC+CBD did not impair recognition.[52] A preliminary study found that CBD in conjunction with another type of drug that acts on the CB1 receptor might work well in addition to the standard antipsychotic drugs, and treat other conditions associated with schizophrenia as well.[84] A large survey study of 1877 individuals found that high-CBD content cannabis types were significantly associated with lower degrees of self-reported psychotic symptoms.[735] A recent study found that CBD may help lower psychotic symptoms by preventing the degradation of an endogenous cannabinoid, anandamide, high levels of which are associated with fewer psychotic symptoms.[63]

Additional Schizophrenia resources:
American Psychiatric Association:
www.psychiatry.org
American Psychological Association: apa.org
Brain and Behavior Research Foundation: bbrfoundation.org
National Alliance for the Mentally Ill: www.nami.org
National Institute of Mental Health: www.nih.gov
Schizophrenia.com: schizophrenia.com
World Health Organization:
www.who.int

Sickle cell disease

Sickle cell disease encompasses a group of inherited red blood cell dis-orders. These cells become hard and sticky, and are shaped to look like a sickle (a farm tool). Sickled cells have a short life span, which causes a shortage of red blood cells, and they tend to get stuck in small blood vessels because of their shape, clogging the flow of blood and causing pain, infection, acute chest syndrome, and stroke. Sickle cell disease is inherited when a person receives a sickle cell gene variant from each person. Sickle cell disease can only be cured by a bone marrow or stem cell transplant, two procedures that are very risky. The CDC reports that sickle cell disease has varied manifestations depending on the person, and thus symptoms, complications and treatments differ. Symptoms include swelling in hands and feet, and pain from stuck blood vessels, which are usually treated by pain medication and fluid increase. Anemia is a common complication that can be treated by blood transfusions, but this has its own associated serious complications. Infections are common and can be prevented with vaccines and antibiotics. Acute chest syndrome is similar to pneumonia and is treated with medication, oxygen, and sometimes blood transfusions. Splenic sequestration occurs when sickled cells get trapped in the spleen and cause it to enlarge. This can be life threatening and is usually treated with a blood transfusion, but may also require the spleen to be removed. Vision loss, leg ulcers, stroke, pulmonary embolism, deep vein thrombosis, and damage to other body organs are also possible complications. The CDC reports that about 90,000 to 100,000 Americans are affected by sickle cell disease, and that it is more common in African Americans or Blacks.

A survey study of 86 young adults with sickle cell disease found that 36% used cannabis to relieve pain, induce relaxation, or relieve anxiety and depression associated with the disease.[615] A longitudinal study of sickle cell disease found that, although patients might use it to relieve chronic pain and other symptoms, it did not affect clinical severity of the disease.[809]

Additional Sickle cell disease resources:
American Sickle Cell Anemia Association: www.ascaa.org
American Society of Hematology: www.hematology.org
March of Dimes: www.marchofdimes.org
National Heart, Lung, and Blood Institute: www.nhlbi.nih.gov
Sickle Cell Disease Association of America: www.sicklecelldisease.org
Sickle Cell Information Center: scinfo.org--
United States Centers for Disease Control and Prevention: www.cdc.gov
World Health Organization: www.who.int

Sleep disorders

Sleep is an important part of daily life, and research shows that insufficient sleep is linked to development of chronic adverse conditions. The CDC reports that insufficient sleep is linked to increased risk of Type 2 diabetes, cardiovascular disease, obesity, and depression, for example. The National Heart, Lung, and Blood Institute provides a chart of recommended hours of sleep for humans per day for adults, around 7-8 hours is advised, while infants, children, and teens need more. Sleep disorders range from excessive sleepiness to inability to sleep. The CDC details 4 major sleep disorders, briefly summarized here.

- *Insomnia* can take various forms, but is characterized by an inability to initiate or maintain sleep. It may be a disorder in its own right, or may be a side effect of other conditions or treatments for them.

- *Restless legs syndrome* interrupts sleep through its unpleasant sensations caused in the legs. It is relieved by leg movement, which of courses makes falling asleep difficult. Restless leg syndrome has been associated with dopamine abnormalities.

- *Sleep apnea* is a condition in which a person gasps, snorts, or snores, interrupting their sleep. It can cause excessive daytime sleepiness because the nighttime sleep is not restful.

- *Narcolepsy* is a condition of excessive daytime sleepiness, including episodes of irresistible sleep and sudden muscle weakness.

In Chapter 3 we discussed the verified benefits of cannabis for sleep disturbances related to ALS, arthritis, Crohn's disease, epilepsy, Huntington's disease, Parkinson's disease, and PTSD, and in this chapter we have discussed how cannabis can benefit sleep issues related to alcohol dependence, anxiety disorders, attention deficit hyperactivity disorder, bipolar disorder, bladder dysfunction, depression, and chronic prostatitis/pelvic pain syndrome. [33, 53, 227, 239, 474, 478, 500, 529, 593, 605, 617, 618, 630, 665] A study of THC in squirrel monkeys found that it increased drowsiness.[817] A study of healthy young adults found that a 15 mg dose of THC induced sleepiness (although also impaired memory), while 15 mg of CBD had alerting properties and counteracted the residual sleepiness of the THC.[167] Individuals who use cannabis report that sleep quality deteriorates after discontinuation of use,[811] but poor sleep quality before cessation of cannabis also is associated with relapse of cannabis use.[810] Tolerance to the sedating effects of THC may also occur with chronic, high-dose usag.[813] Because of its wakefulness properties, CBD may prove useful in sleep disorders characterized by excessive sleepiness. In laboratory rats, CBD increases wakefulness.[814, 816] Injection of CBD increases extracellular levels of adenosine (a sleep-inducing molecule),[812] and increases total sleep time, but also increases the amount of time it takes to fall asleep during light hours[34], as well as increasing dopamine levels (a wake-inducing molecule).[815]

Additional Sleep disorders resources:
Anxiety Disorders Association of America: www.adaa.org
National Sleep Foundation: sleepfoundation.org
United States Centers for Disease Control and Prevention: www.cdc.gov

Transmissible spongiform encephalopathies

Transmissible spongiform encephalopathies are also known as prion diseases, after the abnormal protein that causes them. The prion is a misfolded protein that can propagate itself by causing conformational changes in other, normally folded proteins in the brain. Upon contact with the normally folded proteins, the prion induces the normal protein to misfold as well. This new misfolded protein, now also a prion, then causes misfolding of other normal proteins it touches, and so on. A chain reaction is created in which the normal proteins are induced by the prions to reconfigure, and misfolded masses of proteins and holes in the brain appear. This characteristic "spongy" appearance gave the diseases their name.

Spongiform encephalopathies are fatal diseases that can occur in a variety of mammal species, including humans. Scrapie occurs in sheep and goats, and has been known in Europe for centuries. Chronic wasting disease, for example, was discovered in Colorado in deer in the 1960s. In addition, the CDC also lists a transmissible mink encephalopathy, feline spongiform encephalopathy, and ungulate spongiform encephalopathy.

Bovine spongiform encephalopathy is also known as "mad cow" disease, and an epidemic that occurred in Britain in the 1980s helped scientists discover the link between the human and animal prion diseases.

Spongiform encephalopathies can be transmitted, can occur sporadically, with no predictable indicator or risk factor, or they can more rarely occur as an inherited disease due to a genetic defect. Researchers have now found dozens of mutations in the gene that makes the prion protein, which can cause Creutzfeldt-Jakob disease (CJD), fatal familial insomnia, Gerstmann-Straussler-Scheinker disease, and kuru. Fortunately, these are very, very rare in humans. The common characteristics of prion diseases are sleep disturbances, personality changes, problems with memory and vision, weakness, muscle atrophy, and lack of coordination. As the disease spreads, the brain becomes more affected, and ultimately death is the outcome. There is currently no known cure for prion diseases.

The known neuroprotective effects of cannabis prompted a group of researchers to assay cannabinoids for their ability to affect accumulation of prions in cell cultures and in mice. CBD inhibited prion accumulation in cells that were infected with sheep and mouse prion strains, and also increased the survival of mice infected with scrapie. Although it is unclear exactly how CBD inhibited the prions, it is thought to be a potential therapeutic agent against prions.[24]

A

Acute: of sudden onset and short duration.

Adipose tissue: one of the main types of connective tissue, composed of fat cells.

Adipogenesis: creation of adipose cells (fat cells).

Analgesic: a substance that causes relief from pain.

Anemia: decrease of number of red blood cells or decrease of amount of hemoglobin in the blood. Hemoglobin is the protein that carries oxygen to the lungs.

Angiogenesis: the process through which new blood vessels form.

Anorexia: a lack of appetite for food.

Anti-microbial: a substance that kills microorganisms or that inhibits growth of microorganisms. Microorganisms are bacteria, fungi, and viruses.

Anti-oxidant: a substance that inhibits oxidation of molecules. Oxidation is a chemical reaction that may cause some types of cell damage.

Anti-prion: a misfolded protein that can cause a chain reaction of misfolding in other proteins that it contacts.

Anti-proliferative: a substance that prevents or slows the growth of cells, usually referring to tumors.

Anti-retroviral drug: a drug that inhibits or kills retroviruses. Retroviruses work by inserting their genetic material into a host cell and then using an enzyme called reverse transcriptase to integrate their genetic material into the host's genetic material. In this way, the host's own cellular processes express the virus's genetic material, making more viruses that can then go on to infect more cells.

Anti-tussive: a substance that relieves coughing.

Anxiogenic: something that induces anxiety.

Anxiolytic: something that reduces anxiety.

Apoptosis: programmed cell death.

Autoimmune disorder: A condition in which the body's own immune system mistakenly attacks healthy body tissues.

C

Cardiomyopathy: disease of the heart muscle.

Chorea: an abnormal involuntary movement disorder.

Chronic: progressive development and of extend duration.

Cirrhosis: scarring of the liver.

Cognitive: relating to mental abilities and processes such as knowledge, attention, memory, judgment, evaluation, perception, creativity.

Convulsant: something that induces seizures.

D

Dioecious: a plant that has the male and female reproductive organs in separate individuals.

Dystonia: a neurological disorder characterized by involuntary muscle contractions and repetitive movements or abnormal postures.

E

Efficacy: the capacity to produce a desired or intended result or effect.

Embryotoxic: harmful to the developing embryo.

Emetic: a substance that causes nausea and vomiting.

Endogenous: a substance or condition originating from within an organism.

Enterotoxigenic: a substance causing toxicity in the intestines. Enterotoxins are secreted by many bacterial species.

Epidemiological: of the science that studies the patterns, causes, and effects of health and disease in populations.

Excitotoxicity: a process in which nerve cells are damaged and killed by overstimulation of receptors.

Exogenous: a substance or condition originating from outside of an organism.

G

Glial cells: cells of the central nervous system that are not neurons – they do not conduct electrical impulses, but instead surround the neurons and provide support and insulation between them.

Glioma: a type of brain or spine tumor that arises from glial cells.

H

Hematopoietic: the cells that will give rise to the body's blood cells.

Hepatic: involving the liver.

Hyperalgesic: causing increased sensitivity to pain.

Hypertension: high pressure – high blood pressure, or high pressure inside the eye.

Hypoglycemia: low blood sugar.

Hypotension: low pressure-low blood pressure.

I

Immunodeficiency: a state in which the immune system is deficient, i.e., it is not able to perform its normal functions (such as fighting against infectious organisms).

Immunomodulatory: something that modulates or regulates some part of the immune system.

Immunosuppressive: something that suppresses some part of the immune system.

In vitro: literally, the Latin means in glass. In vitro studies are those performed outside the body, for example, in a test tube or in a cell culture.

Inflammation: a natural biological response to damage or invasion by foreign substances in which the body's immune cells and chemicals are released to the blood or affected tissue to fight against the injury or foreign substance.

Insulitis: inflammation of the islets of Langerhans regions of the pancreas. These regions have cells that make insulin.

Intractable: difficult to control. Intractable pain is pain that is not easily managed, if at all.

J

Jaundice: a condition in which too much of a yellow chemical called bilirubin that is normally present in your red blood cells builds up and makes the skin and whites of the eyes turn yellow. The bilirubin builds up because the liver cannot handle the red cells that are breaking down.

L

Lesion: a damaged portion of a tissue, such as a wound, ulcer, abscess, or tumor.

Lipid: naturally occurring fats, waxes, and certain other molecules that are not soluble in water.

Lymphedema: blockage of the lymphatic system (part of the immune system) that causes fluid buildup leading to swelling.

M

Macroparasites: parasites are organisms that benefit by living in or on another organism that is harmed by the relationship. A macroparasite is one large enough to be seen with the naked eye, such as a pin worm or tape worm.

Meta-analysis: a statistical analysis of several independent experiments to test the data for statistical significance.

Metastatis: the spread of cancer cells from one part of the body to another.

Microparasites: parasites are organisms that benefit by living in or on another organism that is harmed by the relationship. A microparasite is one so small that it must be seen with a microscope, such as a virus.

Mitochondria: an organelle inside of cells that make energy for the cell to use. Mitochondria have their own genome, and thus there can be genetic mitochondrial diseases.

Monoecious: a plant that has the male and female reproductive organs in the same individual.

N

Neurocognitive: cognitive means relating to mental abilities and processes such as knowledge, attention, memory, judgment, evaluation, perception, creativity. Neurocognitive refers to the physical components (such as nerves or brain matter) underlying cognition.

Neurodegenerative: a process of the loss of structure or function of nerve cells, including nerve cell death.

Neurological: pertaining to the nervous system, i.e., the brain, spinal cord, and nerves.

Neuroimaging: using techniques to either directly or indirectly make an image of the structure or function of the nervous system. There are several neuroimaging techniques; an example of one is magnetic resonance imaging (MRI) which uses magnetic fields and radio waves to produce images of brain structures.

Neuron: a nerve cell.

Neuropathic: an abnormal or diseased condition of the nervous system.

Neuroprotective: something that protects the nervous system or its components.

Neurotransmitter: chemicals in the body that transmit signals from one nerve cell to another.

Nociceptive: relating to a sensation from the stimulation of nerve cells that is generally perceived as pain.

O

Orexigenic: something that stimulates the appetite.

Oxidative stress: an imbalance between certain types of molecules in the body and the body's ability to detoxify the molecules or repair the damage caused.

P

Peripheral nerves: those outside the brain and spinal cord.

Physical therapy: broadly speaking, is a type of rehabilitative intervention in which a trained professional uses physical (non-chemical) methods and treatments to reduce pain and restore mobility.

Phytochemical: chemicals that come from plants.

Placebo: a harmless or inactive substance that is used as a control when testing a drug.

Polycyclic: having multiple cycles.

Psychoactive: having the property of changing brain function and altering perception.

Psychotherapy: broadly speaking, psychotherapy is the treatment of mental health problems by talking to a trained mental health worker who has access to techniques that can help the patient handle the problems or even resolve them.

Psychotic: characterized by abnormal thinking and perceptions. Loss of touch with reality.

R

Refractory: resistant or unmanageable. Refractory pain is pain that is resistant to treatment.

Remission: in terms of disease, a condition in which signs and symptoms of the disease have disappeared, although the disease may still be present in the body.

S

Somnolence: drowsiness or sleepiness.

T

Tachycardia: faster than normal heartbeat.

Toxin: a poisonous substance that can harm the body.

V

Vasoconstriction: narrowing of the blood vessels.

REFERENCES

1. Russo E, et al. (2008) Phytochemical and genetic analyses of ancient cannabis from Central Asia. *J Exp Bot* 59(15):4171–4182.

2. Van Bakel H, et al. (2011) The draft genome and transcriptome of Cannabis sativa. *Genome Biol* 12:R102.

3. Russo E (2007) History of cannabis and its preparations in saga, science, and sobriquet. *Chem Biodivers* 4:1614–1648.

4. Pertwee RG (2006) Cannabinoid pharmacology: the first 66 years. *Br J Pharmacol* 147 Suppl :S163–71.

5. Bostwick JM (2012) Blurred boundaries: the therapeutics and politics of medical marijuana. *Mayo Clin Proc* 87(2):172–86.

6. Zias J, et al. (1993) Early medical use of cannabis. *Nature* 363(6426):215.

7. Clark PA, Capuzzi K, Fick C (2011) Medical marijuana: medical necessity versus political agenda. *Med Sci Monit* 17(12):RA249–61.

8. Mikuriya T (2004) Cannabis as a substitute for alcohol: a harm-reduction approach. *J cannabis Ther* 4(1):79–93.

9. Williams E, Himmelsbach C, Wikler A, Ruble D, Lloyd Jr B (1946) Studies on marihuana and pyrahexyl compound. *Public Health Rep* 61(29):1059–1083.

10. Brenneisen R (2007) Chemistry and analysis of phytocannabinoids and other Cannabis constituents. *Marijuana and the Cannabinoids*, ed ElSohly M (Humana Press, Totowa, NJ), pp 17–49.

11. Giacoppo S, Mandolino G, Galuppo M, Bramanti P, Mazzon E (2014) Cannabinoids: new promising agents in the treatment of neurological diseases. *Molecules* 19(11):18781–816.

12. Radwan MM, et al. (2009) Biologically active cannabinoids from high-potency Cannabis sativa. *J Nat Prod* 72(5):906–11.

13. Robson P (2001) Therapeutic aspects of cannabis and cannabinoids. *Br J Psychiatry* 178:107–115.

14. Buchweitz JP, Karmaus PWF, Williams KJ, Harkema JR, Kaminski NE (2008) Targeted deletion of cannabinoid receptors CB1 and CB2 produced enhanced inflammatory responses to influenza A/PR/8/34 in the absence and presence of Delta9-tetrahydrocannabinol. *J Leukoc Biol* 83(3):785–96.

15. Avraham Y, et al. (2011) Cannabidiol improves brain and liver function in a fulminant hepatic failure-induced model of hepatic encephalopathy in mice. *Br J Pharmacol* 162(7):1650–8.

16. De Petrocellis L, et al. (2013) Non-THC cannabinoids counteract prostate carcinoma growth in vitro and in vivo: pro-apoptotic effects and underlying mechanisms. *Br J Pharmacol* 168(1):79–102.

17. Romano B, et al. (2013) The cannabinoid TRPA1 agonist cannabichromene inhibits nitric oxide production in macrophages and ameliorates murine colitis. *Br J Pharmacol* 169(1):213–29.

18. Izzo AA, et al. (2012) Inhibitory effect of cannabichromene, a major non-psychotropic cannabinoid extracted from Cannabis sativa, on inflammation-induced hypermotility in mice. *Br J Pharmacol* 166(4):1444–60.

19. Klein T, Cabral G (2006) Cannabinoid-induced immunesuppression and modulation of antigen-presenting cells. *J Neuroimmune Pharmacol* 1(1):50–64.

20. Appendino G, et al. (2008) Antibacterial cannabinoids from Cannabis sativa: a structure-activity study. *J Nat Prod* 71(8):1427–30.

21. Nagarkatti P, Pandey R, Rieder SA, Hegde VL, Nagarkatti M (2009) Cannabinoids as novel anti-inflammatory drugs. *Future Med Chem* 1(7):1333–49.

22. Hampson AJ, Grimaldi M, Axelrod J, Wink D (1998) Cannabidiol and (-)Delta9-tetrahydrocannabinol are neuroprotective antioxidants. *Proc Natl Acad Sci U S A* 95(14):8268–73.

23. Fride E, Ponde D, Breuer A, Hanus L (2005) Peripheral, but not central effects of cannabidiol derivatives: mediation by CB(1) and unidentified receptors. *Neuropharmacology* 48(8):1117–29.

24. Dirikoc S, Priola SA, Marella M, Zsürger N, Chabry J (2007) Nonpsychoactive cannabidiol prevents prion accumulation and protects neurons against prion toxicity. *J Neurosci* 27(36):9537–44.

25. Ahrens J, et al. (2009) The nonpsychotropic cannabinoid cannabidiol modulates and directly activates alpha-1 and alpha-1-Beta glycine receptor function. *Pharmacology* 83(4):217–22.

26. Almeida V, et al. (2013) Cannabidiol exhibits anxiolytic but not antipsychotic property evaluated in the social interaction test. *Prog Neuropsychopharmacol Biol Psychiatry* 41:30–5.

27. Aviello G, et al. (2012) Chemopreventive effect of the non-psychotropic phytocannabinoid cannabidiol on experimental colon cancer. *J Mol Med (Berl)* 90(8):925–34.

28. Borrelli F, et al. (2009) Cannabidiol, a safe and non-psychotropic ingredient of the marijuana plant Cannabis sativa, is protective in a murine model of colitis. *J Mol Med (Berl)* 87(11):1111–21.

29. Campos AC, et al. (2013) Involvement of serotonin-mediated neurotransmission in the dorsal periaqueductal gray matter on cannabidiol chronic effects in panic-like responses in rats. *Psychopharmacology (Berl)* 226(1):13–24.

30. Campos AC, Ferreira FR, Guimarães FS (2012) Cannabidiol blocks long-lasting behavioral consequences of predator threat stress: possible involvement of 5HT1A receptors. *J Psychiatr Res* 46(11):1501–10.

31. Capasso R, et al. (2008) Cannabidiol, extracted from Cannabis sativa, selectively inhibits inflammatory hypermotility in mice. *Br J Pharmacol* 154(5):1001–8.

32. Carlini EA, Mechoulam R, Lander N (1975) Anticonvulsant activity of four oxygenated cannabidiol derivatives. *Res Commun Chem Pathol Pharmacol* 12(1):1–15.

33. Chagas MHN, et al. (2014) Cannabidiol can improve complex sleep-related behaviours associated with rapid eye movement sleep behaviour disorder in Parkinson's disease patients: a case series. *J Clin Pharm Ther* 39(5):564–6.

34. Chagas MHN, et al. (2013) Effects of acute systemic administration of cannabidiol on sleep-wake cycle in rats. *J Psychopharmacol* 27(3):312–6.

35. Chagas MHN, et al. (2014) Effects of cannabidiol in the treatment of patients with Parkinson's disease: an exploratory double-blind trial. *J Psychopharmacol* 28(11):1088–98.

36. Chesher GB, Jackson DM, Malor RM (1975) Interaction of delta9-tetrahydrocannabinol and cannabidiol with phenobarbitone in protecting mice from electrically induced convulsions. *J Pharm Pharmacol* 27(8):608–9.

37. Consroe P, Martin P, Eisenstein D (1977) Anticonvulsant drug antagonism of delta9tetrahydrocannabinol-induced seizures in rabbits. *Res Commun Chem Pathol Pharmacol* 16(1):1–13.

38. Consroe P, Sandyk R, Snider SR (1986) Open label evaluation of cannabidiol in dystonic movement disorders. *Int J Neurosci* 30(4):277–82.

39. Costa B, et al. (2004) Oral anti-inflammatory activity of cannabidiol, a non-psychoactive constituent of cannabis, in acute carrageenan-induced inflammation in the rat paw. *Naunyn Schmiedebergs Arch Pharmacol* 369(3):294–9.

40. Costa B, Trovato AE, Comelli F, Giagnoni G, Colleoni M (2007) The non-psychoactive cannabis constituent cannabidiol is an orally effective therapeutic agent in rat chronic inflammatory and neuropathic pain. *Eur J Pharmacol* 556(1-3):75–83.

41. Crippa J, et al. (2011) Neural basis of anxiolytic effects of cannabidiol (CBD) in generalized social anxiety disorder: a preliminary report. *J Psychopharmacol* 25(1):121–130.

42. Cunha JM, et al. (1980) Chronic administration of cannabidiol to healthy volunteers and epileptic patients. *Pharmacology* 21(3):175–85.

43. De Campos AC, Brant F, Miranda AS, Machado FS, Teixeira AL (2015) Cannabidiol increases survival and promotes rescue of cognitive function in a murine model of cerebral malaria. *Neuroscience.*

44. Esposito G, et al. (2007) Cannabidiol in vivo blunts beta-amyloid induced neuroinflammation by suppressing IL-1beta and iNOS expression. *Br J Pharmacol* 151(8):1272–9.

45. Fouad AA, Al-Mulhim AS, Gomaa W (2013) Protective effect of cannabidiol against cadmium hepatotoxicity in rats. *J Trace Elem Med Biol* 27(4):355–63.

46. Fouad AA, Al-Mulhim AS, Jresat I (2012) Cannabidiol treatment ameliorates ischemia/reperfusion renal injury in rats. *Life Sci* 91(7-8):284–92.

47. Gomes F V, et al. (2014) Cannabidiol Attenuates Sensorimotor Gating Disruption and Molecular Changes Induced by Chronic Antagonism of NMDA receptors in Mice. *Int J Neuropsychopharmacol.*

48. Gomes F V, et al. (2015) Decreased glial reactivity could be involved in the antipsychotic-like effect of cannabidiol. *Schizophr Res.*

49. Hao E, et al. (2015) Cannabidiol protects against doxorubicin-induced cardiomyopathy by modulating mitochondrial function and biogenesis. *Mol Med.*

50. Hayakawa K, et al. (2008) Cannabidiol prevents a post-ischemic injury progressively induced by cerebral ischemia via a high-mobility group box1-inhibiting mechanism. *Neuropharmacology* 55(8):1280–6.

51. Hernán Pérez de la Ossa D, et al. (2013) Local delivery of cannabinoid-loaded microparticles inhibits tumor growth in a murine xenograft model of glioblastoma multiforme. *PLoS One* 8(1):e54795.

52. Hindocha C, et al. (2014) Acute effects of delta-9-tetrahydrocannabinol, cannabidiol and their combination on facial emotion recognition: A randomised, double-blind, placebo-controlled study in cannabis users. *Eur Neuropsychopharmacol.*

53. Hsiao Y-T, Yi P-L, Li C-L, Chang F-C (2012) Effect of cannabidiol on sleep disruption induced by the repeated combination tests consisting of open field and elevated plus-maze in rats. *Neuropharmacology* 62(1):373–84.

54. Ignatowska-Jankowska B, Jankowski M, Glac W, Swiergel AH (2009) Cannabidiol-induced lymphopenia does not involve NKT and NK cells. *J Physiol Pharmacol* 60 Suppl 3:99–103.

55. Iseger TA, Bossong MG (2015) A systematic review of the antipsychotic properties of cannabidiol in humans. *Schizophr Res.*

56. Jamontt JM, Molleman A, Pertwee RG, Parsons ME (2010) The effects of Delta-tetrahydrocannabinol and cannabidiol alone and in combination on damage, inflammation and in vitro motility disturbances in rat colitis. *Br J Pharmacol* 160(3):712–23.

57. Jones NA, et al. (2012) Cannabidiol exerts anti-convulsant effects in animal models of temporal lobe and partial seizures. *Seizure* 21(5):344–52.

58. Kozela E, et al. (2011) Cannabidiol inhibits pathogenic T cells, decreases spinal microglial activation and ameliorates multiple sclerosis-like disease in C57BL/6 mice. *Br J Pharmacol* 163(7):1507–19.

59. Kozela E, et al. (2013) Cannabinoids decrease the th17 inflammatory autoimmune phenotype. *J Neuroimmune Pharmacol* 8(5):1265–76.

60. Kwiatkowska M, Parker LA, Burton P, Mechoulam R (2004) A comparative analysis of the potential of cannabinoids and ondansetron to suppress cisplatin-induced emesis in the Suncus murinus (house musk shrew). *Psychopharmacology (Berl)* 174(2):254–9.

61. Lastres-Becker I, Molina-Holgado F, Ramos JA, Mechoulam R, Fernández-Ruiz J Cannabinoids provide neuroprotection against 6-hydroxydopamine toxicity in vivo and in vitro: relevance to Parkinson's disease. *Neurobiol Dis* 19(1-2):96–107.

62. Levin R, et al. (2012) Antipsychotic profile of cannabidiol and rimonabant in an animal model of emotional context processing in schizophrenia. *Curr Pharm Des* 18(32):4960–5.

63. Leweke FM, et al. (2012) Cannabidiol enhances anandamide signaling and alleviates psychotic symptoms of schizophrenia. *Transl Psychiatry* 2:e94.

64. Ligresti A, et al. (2006) Antitumor activity of plant cannabinoids with emphasis on the effect of cannabidiol on human breast carcinoma. *J Pharmacol Exp Ther* 318(3):1375–87.

65. Long LE, et al. (2010) A behavioural comparison of acute and chronic Delta9-tetrahydrocannabinol and cannabidiol in C57BL/6JArc mice. *Int J Neuropsychopharmacol* 13(7):861–76.

66. Magen I, et al. (2009) Cannabidiol ameliorates cognitive and motor impairments in mice with bile duct ligation. *J Hepatol* 51(3):528–34.

67. Malfait A, et al. (2000) The nonpsychoactive cannabis constituent cannabidiol is an oral anti-arthritic therapeutic in murine collagen-induced arthritis. *Proc Natl Acad Sci USA* 97(17):9561–9566.

68. Marcu JP, et al. (2010) Cannabidiol enhances the inhibitory effects of delta9-tetrahydrocannabinol on human glioblastoma cell proliferation and survival. *Mol Cancer Ther* 9(1):180–9.

69. Martín-Moreno AM, et al. (2011) Cannabidiol and other cannabinoids reduce microglial activation in vitro and in vivo: relevance to Alzheimer's disease. *Mol Pharmacol* 79(6):964–73.

70. Massi P, et al. (2004) Antitumor effects of cannabidiol, a nonpsychoactive cannabinoid, on human glioma cell lines. *J Pharmacol Exp Ther* 308(3):838–45.

71. Mecha M, et al. (2012) Cannabidiol protects oligodendrocyte progenitor cells from inflammation-induced apoptosis by attenuating endoplasmic reticulum stress. *Cell Death Dis* 3:e331.

72. Mecha M, et al. (2013) Cannabidiol provides long-lasting protection against the deleterious effects of inflammation in a viral model of multiple sclerosis: a role for A2A receptors. *Neurobiol Dis* 59:141–50.

73. Moreira FA, Aguiar DC, Guimarães FS (2006) Anxiolytic-like effect of cannabidiol in the rat Vogel conflict test. *Prog Neuropsychopharmacol Biol Psychiatry* 30(8):1466–71.

74. Morgan CJA, et al. (2012) Sub-chronic impact of cannabinoids in street cannabis on cognition, psychotic-like symptoms and psychological well-being. *Psychol Med* 42(2):391–400.

75. Morgan CJA, Curran HV (2008) Effects of cannabidiol on schizophrenia-like symptoms in people who use cannabis. *Br J Psychiatry* 192(4):306–7.

76. Mukhopadhyay P, et al. (2011) Cannabidiol protects against hepatic ischemia/reperfusion injury by attenuating inflammatory signaling and response, oxidative/nitrative stress, and cell death. *Free Radic Biol Med* 50(10):1368–81.

77. Notcutt W, et al. (2004) Initial experiences with medicinal extracts of cannabis for chronic pain: results from 34 "N of 1" studies. *Anaesthesia* 59(5):440–452.

78. Oláh A, et al. (2014) Cannabidiol exerts sebostatic and antiinflammatory effects on human sebocytes. *J Clin Invest* 124(9):3713–24.

79. Parker LA, Kwiatkowska M, Burton P, Mechoulam R (2004) Effect of cannabinoids on lithium-induced vomiting in the Suncus murinus (house musk shrew). *Psychopharmacology (Berl)* 171(2):156–61.

80. Perez M, et al. (2013) Neuroprotection and reduction of glial reaction by cannabidiol treatment after sciatic nerve transection in neonatal rats. *Eur J Neurosci* 38(10):3424–34.

81. Rajesh M, et al. (2010) Cannabidiol attenuates cardiac dysfunction, oxidative stress, fibrosis, and inflammatory and cell death signaling pathways in diabetic cardiomyopathy. *J Am Coll Cardiol* 56(25):2115–25.

82. Ramer R, et al. (2012) Cannabidiol inhibits lung cancer cell invasion and metastasis via intercellular adhesion molecule-1. *FASEB J* 26(4):1535–48.

83. Ren Y, Whittard J, Higuera-Matas A, Morris C V, Hurd YL (2009) Cannabidiol, a nonpsychotropic component of cannabis, inhibits cue-induced heroin seeking and normalizes discrete mesolimbic neuronal disturbances. *J Neurosci* 29(47):14764–9.

84. Robson PJ, Guy GW, Di Marzo V (2014) Cannabinoids and schizophrenia: therapeutic prospects. *Curr Pharm Des* 20(13):2194–204.

85. Rock EM, et al. (2012) Cannabidiol, a non-psychotropic component of cannabis, attenuates vomiting and nausea-like behaviour via indirect agonism of 5-HT(1A) somatodendritic autoreceptors in the dorsal raphe nucleus. *Br J Pharmacol* 165(8):2620–34.

86. Rock EM, Limebeer CL, Mechoulam R, Piomelli D, Parker LA (2008) The effect of cannabidiol and URB597 on conditioned gaping (a model of nausea) elicited by a lithium-paired context in the rat. *Psychopharmacology (Berl)* 196(3):389–95.

87. Romano B, et al. (2014) Inhibition of colon carcinogenesis by a standardized Cannabis sativa extract with high content of cannabidiol. *Phytomedicine* 21(5):631–9.

88. Sagredo O, et al. (2011) Neuroprotective effects of phytocannabinoid-based medicines in experimental models of Huntington's disease. *J Neurosci Res* 89(9):1509–18.

89. Scott KA, Dalgleish AG, Liu WM (2014) The combination of cannabidiol and δ9-tetrahydrocannabinol enhances the anticancer effects of radiation in an orthotopic murine glioma model. *Mol Cancer Ther* 13(12):2955–67.

90. Scuderi C, Steardo L, Esposito G (2014) Cannabidiol promotes amyloid precursor protein ubiquitination and reduction of beta amyloid expression in SHSY5YAPP+ cells through PPARγ involvement. *Phyther Res* 28(7):1007–1013.

91. Shrivastava A, Kuzontkoski PM, Groopman JE, Prasad A (2011) Cannabidiol induces programmed cell death in breast cancer cells by coordinating the cross-talk between apoptosis and autophagy. *Mol Cancer Ther* 10(7):1161–72.

92. Soares V de P, et al. (2010) Intra-dorsal periaqueductal gray administration of cannabidiol blocks panic-like response by activating 5-HT1A receptors. *Behav Brain Res* 213(2):225–9.

93. Srivastava MD, Srivastava BI, Brouhard B (1998) Delta9 tetra-hydrocannabinol and cannabidiol alter cytokine production by human immune cells. *Immunopharmacology* 40(3):179-85.

94. Torres S, et al. (2011) A combined preclinical therapy of cannabinoids and temozolomide against glioma. *Mol Cancer Ther* 10(1):90-103.

95. Ward SJ, Ramirez MD, Neelakantan H, Walker EA (2011) Cannabidiol prevents the development of cold and mechanical allodynia in paclitaxel-treated female C57Bl6 mice. *Anesth Analg* 113(4):947-50.

96. Ward SJ, et al. (2014) Cannabidiol inhibits paclitaxel-induced neuropathic pain through 5-HT(1A) receptors without diminishing nervous system function or chemotherapy efficacy. *Br J Pharmacol* 171(3):636-45.

97. Weiss L, et al. (2006) Cannabidiol lowers incidence of diabetes in non-obese diabetic mice. *Autoimmunity* 39(2):143-51.

98. Xiong W, et al. (2012) Cannabinoids suppress inflammatory and neuropathic pain by targeting α3 glycine receptors. *J Exp Med* 209(6):1121-34.

99. Zanelati T V, Biojone C, Moreira FA, Guimarães FS, Joca SRL (2010) Antidepressant-like effects of cannabidiol in mice: possible involvement of 5-HT1A receptors. *Br J Pharmacol* 159(1):122-8.

100. Zuardi A, et al. (2006) Cannabidiol monotherapy for treatment-resistant schizophrenia. *J Psychopharmacol* 20(5):683-686.

101. Zuardi A, Morais S, Guimaraes F, Mechoulam R (1995) Antipsychotic effect of cannabidiol. *J Clin Psychiatry* 56:485-486.

102. Rock EM, Kopstick RL, Limebeer CL, Parker LA (2013) Tetrahydrocannabinolic acid reduces nausea-induced conditioned gaping in rats and vomiting in Suncus murinus. *Br J Pharmacol* 170(3):641-8.

103. Rock EM, Parker LA (2013) Suppression of lithium chloride-induced conditioned gaping (a model of nausea-induced behaviour) in rats

(using the taste reactivity test) with metoclopramide is enhanced by cannabidiolic acid. *Pharmacol Biochem Behav* 111:84–9.

104. Takeda S, et al. (2012) Cannabidiolic acid, a major cannabinoid in fiber-type cannabis, is an inhibitor of MDA-MB-231 breast cancer cell migration. *Toxicol Lett* 214(3):314–9.

105. Takeda S, et al. (2014) Down-regulation of cyclooxygenase-2 (COX-2) by cannabidiolic acid in human breast cancer cells. *J Toxicol Sci* 39(5):711–6.

106. Hill AJ, et al. (2012) Cannabidivarin is anticonvulsant in mouse and rat. *Br J Pharmacol* 167(8):1629–42.

107. Hill TDM, et al. (2013) Cannabidivarin-rich cannabis extracts are anticonvulsant in mouse and rat via a CB1 receptor-independent mechanism. *Br J Pharmacol* 170(3):679–92.

108. Rock EM, Sticht MA, Duncan M, Stott C, Parker LA (2013) Evaluation of the potential of the phytocannabinoids, cannabidivarin (CBDV) and Δ(9) -tetrahydrocannabivarin (THCV), to produce CB1 receptor inverse agonism symptoms of nausea in rats. *Br J Pharmacol* 170(3):671–8.

109. Cascio MG, Gauson LA, Stevenson LA, Ross RA, Pertwee RG (2010) Evidence that the plant cannabinoid cannabigerol is a highly potent alpha2-adrenoceptor agonist and moderately potent 5HT1A receptor antagonist. *Br J Pharmacol* 159(1):129–41.

110. Baek SH, et al. (1998) Boron trifluoride etherate on silica-A modified Lewis acid reagent (VII). Antitumor activity of cannabigerol against human oral epitheloid carcinoma cells. *Arch Pharm Res* 21(3):353–6.

111. Borrelli F, et al. (2013) Beneficial effect of the non-psychotropic plant cannabinoid cannabigerol on experimental inflammatory bowel disease. *Biochem Pharmacol* 85(9):1306–16.

112. Borrelli F, et al. (2014) Colon carcinogenesis is inhibited by the TRPM8 antagonist cannabigerol, a Cannabis-derived non-psychotropic cannabinoid. *Carcinogenesis* 35(12):2787–97.

113.   Coetzee C, Levendal R-A, van de Venter M, Frost CL (2007) Anticoagulant effects of a Cannabis extract in an obese rat model. *Phytomedicine* 14(5):333–7.

114.   Shook JE, Burks TF (1989) Psychoactive cannabinoids reduce gastrointestinal propulsion and motility in rodents. *J Pharmacol Exp Ther* 249(2):444–9.

115.   Klein TW, Newton CA (2007) Therapeutic potential of cannabinoid-based drugs. *Adv Exp Med Biol* 601:395–413.

116.   Klein TW (2005) Cannabinoid-based drugs as anti-inflammatory therapeutics. *Nat Rev Immunol* 5(5):400–11.

117.   El-Alfy AT, et al. (2010) Antidepressant-like effect of delta9-tetrahydrocannabinol and other cannabinoids isolated from Cannabis sativa L. *Pharmacol Biochem Behav* 95(4):434–42.

118.   Wiley JL, et al. (2005) CB1 cannabinoid receptor-mediated modulation of food intake in mice. *Br J Pharmacol* 145(3):293–300.

119.   Sanchez-Duffhues G, et al. (2008) Denbinobin, a naturally occurring 1,4-phenanthrenequinone, inhibits HIV-1 replication through an NF-kappaB-dependent pathway. *Biochem Pharmacol* 76(10):1240–1250.

120.   Abrahamov A, Mechoulam R (1995) An efficient new cannabinoid antiemetic in pediatric oncology. *Life Sci* 56(23-24):2097–102.

121.   Birmingham MK (1973) Reduction by 9-tetrahydrocannabinol in the blood pressure of hypertensive rats bearing regenerated adrenal glands. *Br J Pharmacol* 48(1):169–71.

122.   Blázquez C, et al. (2008) Down-regulation of tissue inhibitor of metalloproteinases-1 in gliomas: a new marker of cannabinoid antitumoral activity? *Neuropharmacology* 54(1):235–43.

123.   Blázquez C, et al. (2003) Inhibition of tumor angiogenesis by cannabinoids. *FASEB J* 17(3):529–31.

124.   Blázquez C, et al. (2008) Cannabinoids inhibit glioma cell invasion by down-regulating matrix metalloproteinase-2 expression. *Cancer Res* 68(6):1945–52.

125. Blázquez C, et al. (2004) Cannabinoids inhibit the vascular endothelial growth factor pathway in gliomas. *Cancer Res* 64(16):5617–23.

126. Caffarel MM, Sarrió D, Palacios J, Guzmán M, Sánchez C (2006) Delta9-tetrahydrocannabinol inhibits cell cycle progression in human breast cancer cells through Cdc2 regulation. *Cancer Res* 66(13):6615–21.

127. Chandra LC, et al. (2015) Chronic Administration of Δ9-Tetrahydrocannabinol Induces Intestinal Anti-Inflammatory MicroRNA Expression during Acute Simian Immunodeficiency Virus Infection of Rhesus Macaques. *J Virol* 89(2):1168–81.

128. Chang A, et al. (1979) Delta-9-tetrahydrocannabinol as an antiemetic in cancer patients receiving high-dose methotrexate. *Ann Intern Med* 91:819–824.

129. Chang A, et al. (1981) A prospective evaluation of delta-9-tetrahydrocannabinol as an antiemetic in patients receiving adriamycin and cytoxan chemotherapy. *Cancer* 47:1746–1751.

130. Colls B, Ferry D, Gray A, Harvey V, McQueen E (1980) The antiemetic activity of tetrahydrocanabinol versus metoclopramide and thiethylperazine in patients undergoing cancer chemotherapy. *N Z Med J* 91:449–451.

131. Cooler P, Gregg JM (1977) Effect of delta-9-tetrahydrocannabinol on intraocular pressure in humans. *South Med J* 70(8):951–4.

132. Cotter J (2009) Efficacy of Crude Marijuana and Synthetic Delta-9-Tetrahydrocannabinol as Treatment for Chemotherapy-Induced Nausea and Vomiting: A Systematic Literature Review. *Oncol Nurs Forum* 36(3):345–352.

133. Darmani NA (2001) Delta-9-tetrahydrocannabinol differentially suppresses cisplatin-induced emesis and indices of motor function via cannabinoid CB(1) receptors in the least shrew. *Pharmacol Biochem Behav* 69(1-2):239–49.

134. Darmani NA, Crim JL (2005) Delta-9-tetrahydrocannabinol differentially suppresses emesis versus enhanced locomotor activity

produced by chemically diverse dopamine D2/D3 receptor ago-nists in the least shrew (Cryptotis parva). *Pharmacol Biochem Behav* 80(1):35–44.

135. Dwivedi C, Harbison RD (1975) Anticonvulsant activities of delta-8 and delta-9 tetrahydrocannabinol and uridine. *Toxicol Appl Pharmacol* 31(3):452–8.

136. Ekert H, Waters K, Jurk K, Mobilia J, Loughnan P (1979) Ameriloration of cancer chemotherapy-induced nausea and vomiting by del-ta-9-tetrahydrocannabinol. *Med J Aust* 2:657–659.

137. ElSohly MA, Harland EC, Benigni DA, Waller CW (1984) Cannabinoids in glaucoma II: the effect of different cannabinoids on intraocular pressure of the rabbit. *Curr Eye Res* 3(6):841–50.

138. Eubanks L, et al. (2006) A molecular link between the active com-ponent of marijuana and Alzheimer's disease pathology. *Mol Pharm* 3(6):773–777.

139. Fokos S, Panagis G (2010) Effects of delta9-tetrahydrocannabinol on reward and anxiety in rats exposed to chronic unpredictable stress. *J Psychopharmacol* 24(5):767–77.

140. Frytak S, et al. (1979) Delta-9-tetrahydrocannabinol as an anti-emetics for patients receiving cancer chemotherapy. A com-parison with prochlorperazine and a placebo. *Ann Intern Med* 91:825–830.

141. Gaffal E, Cron M, Glodde N, Tüting T (2013) Anti-inflammatory activity of topical THC in DNFB-mediated mouse allergic con-tact dermatitis independent of CB1 and CB2 receptors. *Allergy* 68(8):994–1000.

142. Galanti G, et al. (2008) Delta 9-tetrahydrocannabinol inhibits cell cycle progression by downregulation of E2F1 in human glioblas-toma multiforme cells. *Acta Oncol* 47(6):1062–70.

143. Galve-Roperh I, et al. (2000) Anti-tumoral action of cannabinoids: involvement of sustained ceramide accumulation and extracellu-lar signal-regulated kinase activation. *Nat Med* 6(3):313–9.

144. Gorka SM, Fitzgerald DA, de Wit H, Phan KL (2014) Cannabinoid Modulation of Amygdala Subregion Functional Connectivity to Social Signals of Threat. *Int J Neuropsychopharmacol* 18(3).

145. Greenwald M, Stitzer M (2000) Antinociceptive, subjective and behavioral effects of smoked marijuana in humans. *Drug Alcohol Depend* 59(3):261–275.

146. Guzmán M, et al. (2006) A pilot clinical study of Delta9-tetrahydrocannabinol in patients with recurrent glioblastoma multiforme. *Br J Cancer* 95(2):197–203.

147. Haroutiunian S, Rosen G, Shouval R, Davidson E (2008) Open-label, add-on study of tetrahydrocannabinol for chronic nonmalignant pain. *J Pain Palliat Care Pharmacother* 22(3):213–217.

148. Hine B, Friedman E, Torrelio M, Gershon S (1975) Tetrahydrocannabinol-attenuated abstinence and induced rotation in morphine-dependent rats: possible involvement of dopamine. *Neuropharmacology* 14(8):607–10.

149. Hine B, Torrelio M, Gershon S (1975) Attenuation of precipitated abstinence in methadone-dependent rats by delta 9-THC. *Psychopharmacol Commun* 1(3):275–83.

150. Hine B, Friedman E, Torrelio M, Gershon S (1975) Morphine-dependent rats: blockade of precipitated abstinence by tetrahydrocannabinol. *Science* 187(4175):443–5.

151. Hornby P, Sharma M (2010) Standardized cannabis in multiple sclerosis: a case report. *Cases J* 3:7.

152. Jabusch H-C, Schneider U, Altenmüller E (2004) Delta9-tetrahydrocannabinol improves motor control in a patient with musician's dystonia. *Mov Disord* 19(8):990–1.

153. Kluin-Nelemans J, NElemans F, Meuwissen Ojat, Maes R (1979) Delta9-tetrahydrocannabinol (THC) as an antiemetic in patients treated with cancer chemotherapy; a double-blind cross-over trial against placeb. *Vet Hum Toxicol* 21:338–340.

154. Lee MC, et al. (2013) Amygdala activity contributes to the dissociative effect of cannabis on pain perception. *Pain* 154(1):124–34.

155. Leelawat S, Leelawat K, Narong S, Matangkasombut O (2010) The dual effects of delta(9)-tetrahydrocannabinol on cholangiocarcinoma cells: anti-invasion activity at low concentration and apoptosis induction at high concentration. *Cancer Invest* 28(4):357–63.

156. Levitt M, Faiman C, Hawks R, Wilson A (1984) Randomized double blind comparison of delta-9-tetrahydroicannabinol (THC) and marijuana as chemotherapy antiemetics. *Proc Am Soc Clin Oncol* 3:91.

157. Levitt M, et al. (1981) Dose vs response of tetrahydroannabinol (THC) vs prochlorperazine as chemotherapy antiemetics. *Proc Am Soc Clin Oncol* 22:422.

158. Liu WM, Scott KA, Shamash J, Joel S, Powles TB (2008) Enhancing the in vitro cytotoxic activity of Delta9-tetrahydrocannabinol in leukemic cells through a combinatorial approach. *Leuk Lymphoma* 49(9):1800–9.

159. Makwana R, Venkatasamy R, Spina D, Page C (2015) THE EFFECT OF PHYTOCANNABINOIDS ON AIRWAY HYPERRESPONSIVENESS, AIRWAY INFLAMMATION AND COUGH. *J Pharmacol Exp Ther*.

160. McAllister SD, et al. (2005) Cannabinoids selectively inhibit proliferation and induce death of cultured human glioblastoma multiforme cells. *J Neurooncol* 74(1):31–40.

161. McCabe M, et al. (1988) Efficacy of tetrahydrocannabinol in patients refractory to standard anti-emetic therapy. *Invest New Drugs* 6:243–246.

162. McCallum RW, et al. (1999) Delta-9-tetrahydrocannabinol delays the gastric emptying of solid food in humans: a double-blind, randomized study. *Aliment Pharmacol Ther* 13(1):77–80.

163. Medveczky MM, Sherwood TA, Klein TW, Friedman H, Medveczky PG (2004) Delta-9 tetrahydrocannabinol (THC) inhibits lytic replication of gamma oncogenic herpesviruses in vitro. *BMC Med* 2:34.

164. Morel LJ, Giros B, Daugé V (2009) Adolescent exposure to chronic delta-9-tetrahydrocannabinol blocks opiate dependence in maternally deprived rats. *Neuropsychopharmacology* 34(11):2469–76.

165.   Naef M, et al. (2003) The analgesic effect of oral delta-9-tetrahy-drocannabinol (THC), morphine, and a THC-morphine combination in healthy subjects under experimental pain conditions. *Pain* 105(1-2):79–88.

166.   Neidhart J, Gagen M, Wilson H, Young D (1981) Comparative trial of the antiemetic effects of THC and haloperidol. *Int J Clin Pharmacol Res* 21:38S–42S.

167.   Nicholson AN, Turner C, Stone BM, Robson PJ (2004) Effect of Delta-9-tetrahydrocannabinol and cannabidiol on nocturnal sleep and early-morning behavior in young adults. *J Clin Psychopharmacol* 24(3):305–13.

168.   Orr L, McKErnan J, Bloome B (1980) Antiemetic effect of tetrahy-drocannabinol. Compared with placebo and prochlorperazine in chemotherapy-associated nausea and emesis. *Arch Intern Med* 140:1431–1433.

169.   Parker LA, Kwiatkowska M, Mechoulam R (2006) Delta-9-tetrahydrocannabinol and cannabidiol, but not ondansetron, interfere with conditioned retching reactions elicited by a lithium-paired context in Suncus murinus: An animal model of anticipatory nausea and vomiting. *Physiol Behav* 87(1):66–71.

170.   Parker LA, et al. (2003) Effects of cannabinoids on lithium-induced conditioned rejection reactions in a rat model of nausea. *Psychopharmacology (Berl)* 166(2):156–62.

171.   Petro DJ, Ellenberger C (1981) Treatment of human spasticity with delta 9-tetrahydrocannabinol. *J Clin Pharmacol* 21(8-9 Suppl):413S–416S.

172.   Powles T, et al. (2005) Cannabis-induced cytotoxicity in leukemic cell lines: the role of the cannabinoid receptors and the MAPK pathway. *Blood* 105(3):1214–21.

173.   Preet A, Ganju RK, Groopman JE (2008) Delta9-Tetrahydrocannabinol inhibits epithelial growth factor-induced lung cancer cell migration in vitro as well as its growth and metastasis in vivo. *Oncogene* 27(3):339–46.

174. Regelson W, Bulter J, Schulz J (1976) A9-tetrahydrocannabinol as an effective antidepressant and appetite-stimulating agent in advanced cancer patients. *Braude, MC, Szara, S, Eds. The Pharmacology of Marijuana. New York: Raven Press.*, pp 763–776.

175. Ruiz L, Miguel A, Díaz-Laviada I (1999) Delta9-tetrahydrocannabinol induces apoptosis in human prostate PC-3 cells via a receptor-independent mechanism. *FEBS Lett* 458(3):400–4.

176. Sallan S, Cronin C, Zelen M, Zinberg N (1980) Antiemetics in patients receiving chemotherapy for cancer. A randomized comparison of delta-9-tetrahydrocannabinol and prochlorperazine. *N Engl J Med* 302:135–138.

177. Sallan SE, Zinberg NE, Frei E (1975) Antiemetic effect of delta-9-tetrahydrocannabinol in patients receiving cancer chemotherapy. *N Engl J Med* 293(16):795–7.

178. Strasser F, et al. (2006) Comparison of orally administered cannabis extract and delta-9-tetrahydrocannabinol in treating patients with cancer-related anorexia-cachexia syndrome: a multicenter, phase III, randomized, double-blind, placebo-controlled clinical trial from the Cannabi. *J Clin Oncol* 24(21):3394–400.

179. Sweet DL, Miller NJ, Weddington W, Senay E, Sushelsky L (1981) delta 9-Tetrahydrocannabinol as an antiemetic for patients receiving cancer chemotherapy. A pilot study. *J Clin Pharmacol* 21(8-9 Suppl):70S–75S.

180. Ten Ham M, Loskota WJ, Lomax P (1975) Acute and chronic effects of beta9-tetrahydrocannabinol on seizures in the gerbil. *Eur J Pharmacol* 31(1):148–52.

181. Tomida I, et al. (2006) Effect of sublingual application of cannabinoids on intraocular pressure: a pilot study. *J Glaucoma* 15(5):349–53.

182. Ungerleider JT, Andrysiak TA, Fairbanks LA, Tesler AS, Parker RG (1984) Tetrahydrocannabinol vs. prochlorperazine. The effects of two antiemetics on patients undergoing radiotherapy. *Radiology* 150(2):598–9.

183. Ungerleider JT, et al. (1982) Cannabis and cancer chemotherapy: a comparison of oral delta-9-THC and prochlorperazine. *Cancer* 50(4):636–45.

184. Ungerleider JT, Andyrsiak T, Fairbanks L, Ellison GW, Myers LW (1987) Delta-9-THC in the treatment of spasticity associated with multiple sclerosis. *Adv Alcohol Subst Abuse* 7(1):39–50.

185. Vara D, et al. (2011) Anti-tumoral action of cannabinoids on hepatocellular carcinoma: role of AMPK-dependent activation of autophagy. *Cell Death Differ* 18(7):1099–111.

186. Wada JA, Wake A, Sato M, Corcoran ME (1975) Antiepileptic and prophylactic effects of tetrahydrocannabinols in amygdaloid kindled cats. *Epilepsia* 16(3):503–10.

187. Wada JA, Osawa T, Corcoran ME (1975) Effects of tetrahydrocannabinols on kindled amygdaloid seizures and photogenic seizures in Senegalese baboons, Papio papio. *Epilepsia* 16(3):439–48.

188. Whyte DA, et al. (2010) Cannabinoids inhibit cellular respiration of human oral cancer cells. *Pharmacology* 85(6):328–35.

189. Williams RB, Ng LK, Lamprecht F, Roth K, Kopin IJ (1973) 9 -Tetrahydrocannabinol: a hypotensive effect in rats. *Psychopharmacologia* 28(3):269–74.

190. Pertwee RG (2008) The diverse CB1 and CB2 receptor pharmacology of three plant cannabinoids: delta9-tetrahydrocannabinol, cannabidiol and delta9-tetrahydrocannabivarin. *Br J Pharmacol* 153(2):199–215.

191. García C, et al. (2011) Symptom-relieving and neuroprotective effects of the phytocannabinoid Δ^9-THCV in animal models of Parkinson's disease. *Br J Pharmacol* 163(7):1495–506.

192. Tudge L, Williams C, Cowen PJ, McCabe C (2014) Neural Effects of Cannabinoid CB1 Neutral Antagonist Tetrahydrocannabivarin (THCv) on Food Reward and Aversion in Healthy Volunteers. *Int J Neuropsychopharmacol*.

193. Russo EB, Merzouki A, Mesa JM, Frey KA, Bach PJ (2004) Cannabis improves night vision: a case study of dark adaptometry and scotopic sensitivity in kif smokers of the Rif mountains of northern Morocco. *J Ethnopharmacol* 93(1):99–104.

194. Kahan M, Srivastava A, Spithoff S, Bromley L (2014) Prescribing smoked cannabis for chronic noncancer pain: Preliminary recommendations. *Can Fam Physician* 60(12):1083–1090.

195. Guindon J, Hohmann AG (2009) The endocannabinoid system and pain. *CNS Neurol Disord Drug Targets* 8(6):403–21.

196. Fine PG, Rosenfeld MJ (2013) The endocannabinoid system, cannabinoids, and pain. *Rambam Maimonides Med J* 4(4):e0022.

197. Russo EB (2008) Clinical endocannabinoid deficiency (CECD): can this concept explain therapeutic benefits of cannabis in migraine, fibromyalgia, irritable bowel syndrome and other treatment-resistant conditions? *Neuro Endocrinol Lett* 29(2):192–200.

198. Alshaarawy O, Anthony JC (2015) Cannabis smoking and serum C-reactive protein: A quantile regressions approach based on NHANES 2005-2010. *Drug Alcohol Depend* 147:203–7.

199. Bhargava HN (1976) Inhibition of naloxone-induced withdrawal in morphine dependent mice by 1-trans-delta9-tetrahydrocannabinol. *Eur J Pharmacol* 36(1):259–62.

200. Labigalini E, Rodrigues LR, Da Silveira DX (1999) Therapeutic use of cannabis by crack addicts in Brazil. *J Psychoactive Drugs* 31(4):451–5.

201. Mikuriya TH (1970) Cannabis substitution. An adjunctive therapeutic tool in the treatment of alcoholism. *Med Times* 98(4):187–91.

202. Raby WN, et al. Intermittent marijuana use is associated with improved retention in naltrexone treatment for opiate-dependence. *Am J Addict* 18(4):301–8.

203. Reiman A (2009) Cannabis as a substitute for alcohol and other drugs. *Harm Reduct J* 6:35.

204. Abrams DI, Couey P, Shade SB, Kelly ME, Benowitz NL (2011) Cannabinoid-opioid interaction in chronic pain. *Clin Pharmacol Ther* 90(6):844–51.

205. Abrams DI, et al. (2007) Cannabis in painful HIV-associated sensory neuropathy: a randomized placebo-controlled trial. *Neurology* 68(7):515–21.

206. Berman J, et al. (2003) Efficacy of two cannabis-based medicinal extracts for relief of central neuropathic pain from brachial plexus avulsion: results of a randomised controlled trial. *Anaesthesia* 58:938.

207. Berman JS, Symonds C, Birch R (2004) Efficacy of two cannabis based medicinal extracts for relief of central neuropathic pain from brachial plexus avulsion: results of a randomised controlled trial. *Pain* 112(3):299–306.

208. Blake DR, Robson P, Ho M, Jubb RW, McCabe CS (2006) Preliminary assessment of the efficacy, tolerability and safety of a cannabis-based medicine (Sativex) in the treatment of pain caused by rheumatoid arthritis. *Rheumatology (Oxford)* 45(1):50–2.

209. Boychuk DG, Goddard G, Mauro G, Orellana MF (2015) The effectiveness of cannabinoids in the management of chronic nonmalignant neuropathic pain: a systematic review. *J oral facial pain headache* 29(1):7–14.

210. Brady CM, et al. (2004) An open-label pilot study of cannabis-based extracts for bladder dysfunction in advanced multiple sclerosis. *Mult Scler* 10(4):425–33.

211. Cardenas DD, Jensen MP (2006) Treatments for chronic pain in persons with spinal cord injury: A survey study. *J Spinal Cord Med* 29(2):109–17.

212. Comelli F, Bettoni I, Colleoni M, Giagnoni G, Costa B (2009) Beneficial effects of a Cannabis sativa extract treatment on diabetes-induced neuropathy and oxidative stress. *Phytother Res* 23(12):1678–84.

213. Comelli F, Giagnoni G, Bettoni I, Colleoni M, Costa B (2008) Antihyperalgesic effect of a Cannabis sativa extract in a rat model of neuropathic pain: mechanisms involved. *Phytother Res* 22(8):1017–24.

214. Conte A, et al. (2009) Cannabinoid-induced effects on the nociceptive system: a neurophysiological study in patients with secondary progressive multiple sclerosis. *Eur J Pain* 13(5):472–477.

215. Cooper ZD, Comer SD, Haney M (2013) Comparison of the analgesic effects of dronabinol and smoked marijuana in daily marijuana smokers. *Neuropsychopharmacology* 38(10):1984–92.

216. Corey-Bloom J, et al. (2012) Smoked cannabis for spasticity in multiple sclerosis: a randomized, placebo-controlled trial. *CMAJ* 184(10):1143–50.

217. Degenhardt L, et al. (2014) Experience of adjunctive cannabis use for chronic non-cancer pain: Findings from the Pain and Opioids IN Treatment (POINT) study. *Drug Alcohol Depend* 147C:144–150.

218. Ellis RJ, et al. (2009) Smoked medicinal cannabis for neuropathic pain in HIV: a randomized, crossover clinical trial. *Neuropsychopharmacology* 34(3):672–80.

219. El-Mallakh R, Brown C (2007) The effect of extreme marijuana use on the long-term course of bipolar I illness: a single case study. *J Psychoactive Drugs* 39(2):201–202.

220. Fiz J, Durán M, Capellà D, Carbonell J, Farré M (2011) Cannabis use in patients with fibromyalgia: effect on symptoms relief and health-related quality of life. *PLoS One* 6(4):e18440.

221. Hesselink JMK, Kopsky DJ (2012) Intractable neuropathic pain due to ulnar nerve entrapment treated with cannabis and ketamine 10%. *J Clin Anesth* 24(1):78–9.

222. Heutink M, Post MWM, Wollaars MM, van Asbeck FWA (2011) Chronic spinal cord injury pain: pharmacological and non-pharmacological treatments and treatment effectiveness. *Disabil Rehabil* 33(5):433–40.

223. Holdcroft A, Maze M, Dore C, Tebbs S, Thompson S (2006) A multi-center dose-escalation study of the analgesic and adverse effects of an oral cannabis extract (Cannador) for postoperative pain management. *Anesthesiology* 105(5):1040–1046.

224. Holdcroft A, et al. (1997) Pain relief with oral cannabinoids in familial Mediterranean fever. *Anaesthesia* 52:483–488.

225. Iskedjian M, Bereza B, Gordon A, Piwko C, Einarson TR (2007) Meta-analysis of cannabis based treatments for neuropathic and multiple sclerosis-related pain. *Curr Med Res Opin* 23(1):17–24.

226. Johnson J, et al. (2010) Multicenter, Double-Blind, Randomized, Placebo-Controlled, Parallel-Group Study of the Efficacy, Safety, and Tolerability of THC:CBD Extract and THC Extract in Patients With Intractable Cancer-Related Pain. *J Pain Symptom Manage* 39(2):167–179.

227. Lotan I, Treves TA, Roditi Y, Djaldetti R (2014) Cannabis (medical marijuana) treatment for motor and non-motor symptoms of Parkinson disease: an open-label observational study. *Clin Neuropharmacol* 37(2):41–4.

228. Lynch M, Clark A (2003) Cannabis reduces opioid dose in the treatment of chronic non-cancer pain. *J Pain Symptom Manage* 25(6):496–498.

229. Lynch ME, Campbell F (2011) Cannabinoids for treatment of chronic non-cancer pain; a systematic review of randomized trials. *Br J Clin Pharmacol* 72(5):735–44.

230. Milstein SL, MacCannell K, Karr G, Clark S (1975) Marijuana-produced changes in pain tolerance. Experienced and non-experienced subjects. *Int Pharmacopsychiatry* 10(3):177–82.

231. Nurmikko T, et al. (2007) Sativex successfully treats neuropathic pain characterised by allodynia: a randomised, double-blind, placebo-controlled clinical trial. *Pain* 133(1-3):210–220.

232. Perras C (2005) Sativex for the management of multiple sclerosis symptoms. *Issues Emerg Health Technol* (72):1–4.

233. Phillips TJC, Cherry CL, Cox S, Marshall SJ, Rice ASC (2010) Pharmacological treatment of painful HIV-associated sensory neuropathy: a systematic review and meta-analysis of randomised controlled trials. *PLoS One* 5(12):e14433.

234. Richards BL, Whittle SL, Buchbinder R (2012) Neuromodulators for pain management in rheumatoid arthritis. *Cochrane database Syst Rev* 1:CD008921.

235. Rog DJ, Nurmikko TJ, Friede T, Young CA (2005) Randomized, controlled trial of cannabis-based medicine in central pain in multiple sclerosis. *Neurology* 65(6):812–9.

236. Rog D, Nurmikko T, Young C (2007) Oromucosal delta-9-tetrahydrocannabinol/cannabidiol for neuropathic pain associated with multiple sclerosis: an uncontrolled, open-label, 2-year extension trial. *Clin Ther* 29(9):2068–2079.

237. Selvarajah D, Gandhi R, Emery CJ, Tesfaye S (2010) Randomized placebo-controlled double-blind clinical trial of cannabis-based medicinal product (Sativex) in painful diabetic neuropathy: depression is a major confounding factor. *Diabetes Care* 33(1):128–30.

238. Storr M, Devlin S, Kaplan GG, Panaccione R, Andrews CN (2014) Cannabis use provides symptom relief in patients with inflammatory bowel disease but is associated with worse disease prognosis in patients with Crohn's disease. *Inflamm Bowel Dis* 20(3):472–80.

239. Ware MA, Gamsa A, Persson J, Fitzcharles M-A (2002) Cannabis for chronic pain: case series and implications for clinicians. *Pain Res Manag* 7(2):95–9.

240. Ware MA, et al. (2010) Smoked cannabis for chronic neuropathic pain: a randomized controlled trial. *CMAJ* 182(14):E694–701.

241. Wilsey B, et al. (2008) A randomized, placebo-controlled, crossover trial of cannabis cigarettes in neuropathic pain. *J Pain* 9(6):506–21.

242. Wilsey B, et al. (2013) Low-dose vaporized cannabis significantly improves neuropathic pain. *J Pain* 14(2):136–48.

243. Tashkin D, Shapiro B, Lee Y, Harper C (1975) Effects of smoked marijuana in experimentally induced asthma. *Am Rev Respir Dis* 112(3):377–386.

244. Consroe PF, Wood GC, Buchsbaum H (1975) Anticonvulsant nature of marihuana smoking. *JAMA* 234(3):306–7.

245. Cox B, ten Ham M, Loskota WJ, Lomax P (1975) The anticonvulsant activity of cannabinoids in seizure sensitive gerbils. *Proc West Pharmacol Soc* 18:154–7.

246. Hegde M, Santos-Sanchez C, Hess CP, Kabir AA, Garcia PA (2012) Seizure exacerbation in two patients with focal epilepsy following marijuana cessation. *Epilepsy Behav* 25(4):563–6.

247. Maa E, Figi P (2014) The case for medical marijuana in epilepsy. *Epilepsia* 55(6):783–6.

248. Mortati K, Dworetzky B, Devinsky O (2007) Marijuana: an effective antiepileptic treatment in partial epilepsy? A case report and review of the literature. *Rev Neurol Dis* 4(2):103–6.

249. Amtmann D, Weydt P, KL J, MP J, GT C (2004) Survey of cannabis use in patients with amyotrophic lateral sclerosis. *Am J Hosp Palliat Care* 21(2):95–104.

250. Bricker JB, et al. (2007) Does occasional cannabis use impact anxiety and depression treatment outcomes?: Results from a randomized effectiveness trial. *Depress Anxiety* 24(6):392–8.

251. Kvitland L, et al. (2015) Continued cannabis use at one year follow up is associated with elevated mood and lower global functioning in bipolar I disorder. *BMC Psychiatry* 15(1):11.

252. Wallace JL, et al. (2013) Pro-resolution, protective and anti-nociceptive effects of a cannabis extract in the rat gastrointestinal tract. *J Physiol Pharmacol* 64(2):167–75.

253. Uribe Roca MC, Micheli F, Viotti R (2005) Cannabis sativa and dystonia secondary to Wilson's disease. *Mov Disord* 20(1):113–5.

254. Ames FR, Cridland JS (1985) The antiemetic effect of Cannabis sativa during cytotoxic therapy. *S Afr Med J* 68(11):780–1.

255.   Machado Rocha FC, Stéfano SC, De Cássia Haiek R, Rosa Oliveira LMQ, Da Silveira DX (2008) Therapeutic use of Cannabis sativa on chemotherapy-induced nausea and vomiting among cancer patients: systematic review and meta-analysis. *Eur J Cancer Care (Engl)* 17(5):431–43.

256.   Adhiyaman V, Arshad S (2014) Cannabis for intractable nausea after bilateral cerebellar stroke. *J Am Geriatr Soc* 62(6):1199.

257.   Merriman AR, Oliak DA (2008) Use of medical marijuana for treatment of severe intractable nausea after laparoscopic Roux-en-Y gastric bypass surgery. *Surg Obes Relat Dis* 4(4):550–1.

258.   Rock EM, Parker LA (2013) Effect of low doses of cannabidiolic acid and ondansetron on LiCl-induced conditioned gaping (a model of nausea-induced behaviour) in rats. *Br J Pharmacol* 169(3):685–92.

259.   Soderpalm A, Schuster A, de Wit H (2001) Antiemetic efficacy of smoked marijuana: subjective and behavioral effects on nausea induced by syrup of ipecac. *Pharmacology* 69(3-4):343–350.

260.   Söderpalm AH, Schuster A, de Wit H (2014) Antiemetic efficacy of smoked marijuana: subjective and behavioral effects on nausea induced by syrup of ipecac. *Pharmacol Biochem Behav* 69(3-4):343–50.

261.   Tramèr MR, et al. (2001) Cannabinoids for control of chemotherapy induced nausea and vomiting: quantitative systematic review. *BMJ* 323(7303):16–21.

262.   Vinciguerra V, Moore T, Brennan E (1988) Inhalation marijuana as an antiemetic for cancer chemotherapy. *N Y State J Med* 88:525–527.

263.   Flom MC, Adams AJ, Jones RT (1975) Marijuana smoking and reduced pressure in human eyes: drug action or epiphenomenon? *Invest Ophthalmol* 14(1):52–5.

264.   Girgih AT, Alashi A, He R, Malomo S, Aluko RE (2014) Preventive and treatment effects of a hemp seed (Cannabis sativa L.) meal protein hydrolysate against high blood pressure in spontaneously hypertensive rats. *Eur J Nutr* 53(5):1237–46.

265.   Merritt JC (1982) Glaucoma, hypertension, and marijuana. *J Natl Med Assoc* 74(8):715–6.

266.   Merritt JC, Crawford WJ, Alexander PC, Anduze AL, Gelbart SS (1980) Effect of marihuana on intraocular and blood pressure in glaucoma. *Ophthalmology* 87(3):222–8.

267.   West ME, Lockhart AB (1978) The treatment of glaucoma using a non-psychoactive preparation of Cannabis sativa. *West Indian Med J* 27(1):16–25.

268.   Tubaro A, et al. (2010) Comparative topical anti-inflammatory activity of cannabinoids and cannabivarins. *Fitoterapia* 81(7):816–9.

269.   Caffarel MM, et al. (2010) Cannabinoids reduce ErbB2-driven breast cancer progression through Akt inhibition. *Mol Cancer* 9:196.

270.   Carracedo A, et al. (2006) Cannabinoids induce apoptosis of pancreatic tumor cells via endoplasmic reticulum stress-related genes. *Cancer Res* 66(13):6748–55.

271.   Foroughi M, Hendson G, Sargent MA, Steinbok P (2011) Spontaneous regression of septum pellucidum/forniceal pilocytic astrocytomas--possible role of Cannabis inhalation. *Childs Nerv Syst* 27(4):671–9.

272.   Ramer R, Fischer S, Haustein M, Manda K, Hinz B (2014) Cannabinoids inhibit angiogenic capacities of endothelial cells via release of tissue inhibitor of matrix metalloproteinases-1 from lung cancer cells. *Biochem Pharmacol* 91(2):202–16.

273.   Rocha FCM, Dos Santos Júnior JG, Stefano SC, da Silveira DX (2014) Systematic review of the literature on clinical and experimental trials on the antitumor effects of cannabinoids in gliomas. *J Neurooncol* 116(1):11–24.

274.   SCOTT KA, SHAH S, DALGLEISH AG, LIU WM (2013) Enhancing the Activity of Cannabidiol and Other Cannabinoids In Vitro Through Modifications to Drug Combinations and Treatment Schedules. *Anticancer Res* 33(10):4373–4380.

275. Singh Y, Bali C (2013) Cannabis extract treatment for terminal acute lymphoblastic leukemia with a Philadelphia chromosome mutation. *Case Rep Oncol* 6(3):585–92.

276. Collin C, Davies P, Mutiboko IK, Ratcliffe S (2007) Randomized controlled trial of cannabis-based medicine in spasticity caused by multiple sclerosis. *Eur J Neurol* 14(3):290–6.

277. Malec J, Harvey RF, Cayner JJ (1982) Cannabis effect on spasticity in spinal cord injury. *Arch Phys Med Rehabil* 63(3):116–8.

278. Meinck HM, Schönle PW, Conrad B (1989) Effect of cannabinoids on spasticity and ataxia in multiple sclerosis. *J Neurol* 236(2):120–2.

279. Novotna A, et al. (2011) A randomized, double-blind, placebo-controlled, parallel-group, enriched-design study of nabiximols* (Sativex(®)), as add-on therapy, in subjects with refractory spasticity caused by multiple sclerosis. *Eur J Neurol* 18(9):1122–1131.

280. Petro D (1980) Marihuana as a therapeutic agent for muscle spasm or spasticity. *Psychosomatics* 21:81–85.

281. Syed YY, McKeage K, Scott LJ (2014) Delta-9-tetrahydrocannabinol/cannabidiol (Sativex®): a review of its use in patients with moderate to severe spasticity due to multiple sclerosis. *Drugs* 74(5):563–78.

282. Vaney C, et al. (2004) Efficacy, safety and tolerability of an orally administered cannabis extract in the treatment of spasticity in patients with multiple sclerosis: a randomized, double-blind, placebo-controlled, crossover study. *Mult Scler* 10(4):417–24.

283. Wade DT, Makela PM, House H, Bateman C, Robson P (2006) Long-term use of a cannabis-based medicine in the treatment of spasticity and other symptoms in multiple sclerosis. *Mult Scler* 12(5):639–45.

284. Wade DT, Makela P, Robson P, House H, Bateman C (2004) Do cannabis-based medicinal extracts have general or specific effects on symptoms in multiple sclerosis? A double-blind, randomized, placebo-controlled study on 160 patients. *Mult Scler* 10(4):434–41.

285. Wade DT, Robson P, House H, Makela P, Aram J (2003) A preliminary controlled study to determine whether whole-plant cannabis extracts can improve intractable neurogenic symptoms. *Clin Rehabil* 17(1):21–9.

286. Milloy M, et al. (2014) High-intensity cannabis use associated with lower plasma human immunodeficiency virus-1 RNA viral load among recently infected people who use injection drugs. *Drug Alcohol Rev* Nov. 11:Doi:10.1111/dar.12223.

287. Cornelius JR, Aizenstein HJ, Hariri AR (2010) Amygdala reactivity is inversely related to level of cannabis use in individuals with comorbid cannabis dependence and major depression. *Addict Behav* 35(6):644–6.

288. Passie T, Emrich HM, Karst M, Brandt SD, Halpern JH (2012) Mitigation of post-traumatic stress symptoms by Cannabis resin: a review of the clinical and neurobiological evidence. *Drug Test Anal* 4(7-8):649–59.

289. Aukema HM, et al. (2011) Distinctive effects of plant protein sources on renal disease progression and associated cardiac hypertrophy in experimental kidney disease. *Mol Nutr Food Res* 55(7):1044–51.

290. Bourque J, et al. (2013) Cannabis abuse is associated with better emotional memory in schizophrenia: a functional magnetic resonance imaging study. *Psychiatry Res* 214(1):24–32.

291. Molina P, et al. (2011) Cannabinoid neuroimmune modulation of SIV disease. *J Neuroimmune Pharmacol* 6(4):516–527.

292. Molina P, et al. (2011) Cannabinoid administration attenuates the progression of simiman immunodeficiency virus. *AIDS Res Hum Retroviruses* 27(6):585–592.

293. Sexton M, et al. (2014) Cannabis use by individuals with multiple sclerosis: effects on specific immune parameters. *Inflammopharmacology* 22(5):295–303.

294. Abood ME, Rizvi G, Sallapudi N, McAllister SD (2001) Activation of the CB1 cannabinoid receptor protects cultured mouse spinal neurons against excitotoxicity. *Neurosci Lett* 309(3):197–201.

295. Aso E, Sánchez-Pla A, Vegas-Lozano E, Maldonado R, Ferrer I (2015) Cannabis-Based Medicine Reduces Multiple Pathological Processes in AβPP/PS1 Mice. *J Alzheimers Dis* 43(3):977–91.

296. Hermann D, et al. (2007) Dorsolateral prefrontal cortex N-acetylaspartate/total creatine (NAA/tCr) loss in male recreational cannabis users. *Biol Psychiatry* 61(11):1281–9.

297. Nguyen BM, et al. (2014) Effect of marijuana use on outcomes in traumatic brain injury. *Am Surg* 80(10):979–83.

298. Pryce G, Riddall DR, Selwood DL, Giovannoni G, Baker D (2014) Neuroprotection in Experimental Autoimmune Encephalomyelitis and Progressive Multiple Sclerosis by Cannabis-Based Cannabinoids. *J Neuroimmune Pharmacol.*

299. Pryce G, et al. (2003) Cannabinoids inhibit neurodegeneration in models of multiple sclerosis. *Brain* 126(Pt 10):2191–202.

300. Raman C, et al. (2004) Amyotrophic lateral sclerosis: Delayed disease progression in ALS mice by treatment with cannabinoid. *Amyotroph Lateral Scler Other Mot Neuron Disord* 5:33–39.

301. Foltin R, Fishman M, Brady J (1986) Behavioral analysis of marijuana effects on food intake in humans. *Pharmacology* 25:577–582.

302. Foltin R, Fishman M, Byrne M (1988) Effects of smoked marijuana on food intake and body weight of humans living in a residential laboratory. *Appetite* 11(1):1–14.

303. Greenberg I, Kuehnle J, Mendelson J, Bernstein J (1976) Effects of marihuana use on body weight and caloric intake in humans. *Psychopharmacol* 49(1):79–84.

304. Haney M, Rabkin J, Gunderson E, Foltin RW (2005) Dronabinol and marijuana in HIV(+) marijuana smokers: acute effects on caloric intake and mood. *Psychopharmacology (Berl)* 181(1):170–8.

305. Haney M, Rabkin J, Gunderson E, Foltin R (2005) Dronabinol and marijuana in HIV(+) marijuana smokers: acute effects on caloric intake and mood. *Psychopharmacol* 181(1):170–178.

306. Mazidi M, et al. (2014) The effect of hydroalcoholic extract of Cannabis Sativa on appetite hormone in rat. *J Complement Integr Med* 11(4):253–7.

307. Naftali T, et al. (2013) Cannabis induces a clinical response in patients with Crohn's disease: a prospective placebo-controlled study. *Clin Gastroenterol Hepatol* 11(10):1276–1280.e1.

308. Le Foll B, Trigo JM, Sharkey KA, Le Strat Y (2013) Cannabis and Δ9-tetrahydrocannabinol (THC) for weight loss? *Med Hypotheses* 80(5):564–7.

309. Le Strat Y, Le Foll B (2011) Obesity and cannabis use: results from 2 representative national surveys. *Am J Epidemiol* 174(8):929–33.

310. Levendal R-A, Schumann D, Donath M, Frost CL (2012) Cannabis exposure associated with weight reduction and β-cell protection in an obese rat model. *Phytomedicine* 19(7):575–82.

311. Ngueta G, Bélanger RE, Laouan-Sidi EA, Lucas M (2015) Cannabis use in relation to obesity and insulin resistance in the inuit population. *Obesity (Silver Spring)* 23(2):290–5.

312. Penner EA, Buettner H, Mittleman MA (2013) The impact of marijuana use on glucose, insulin, and insulin resistance among US adults. *Am J Med* 126(7):583–9.

313. Warren M, Frost-Pineda K, Gold M (2005) Body mass index and marijuana use. *J Addict Dis* 24(3):95–100.

314. Huang DYC, Lanza HI, Anglin MD (2013) Association between adolescent substance use and obesity in young adulthood: a group-based dual trajectory analysis. *Addict Behav* 38(11):2653–60.

315. Muniyappa R, et al. (2013) Metabolic effects of chronic cannabis smoking. *Diabetes Care* 36(8):2415–22.

316. Del Casale A, et al. (2012) Psychosis risk syndrome comorbid with panic attack disorder in a cannabis-abusing patient affected by Arnold-Chiari malformation type I. *Gen Hosp Psychiatry* 34(6):702. e5–7.

317. Thomas H (1996) A community survey of adverse effects of cannabis use. *Drug Alcohol Depend* 42(3):201–7.

318. Zvolensky MJ, et al. (2006) Lifetime associations between cannabis, use, abuse, and dependence and panic attacks in a representative sample. *J Psychiatr Res* 40(6):477–86.

319. Bambico FR, Nguyen N-T, Katz N, Gobbi G (2010) Chronic exposure to cannabinoids during adolescence but not during adulthood impairs emotional behaviour and monoaminergic neurotransmission. *Neurobiol Dis* 37(3):641–55.

320. Dannon PN, Lowengrub K, Amiaz R, Grunhaus L, Kotler M (2004) Comorbid cannabis use and panic disorder: short term and long term follow-up study. *Hum Psychopharmacol* 19(2):97–101.

321. Ströhle A, Müller M, Rupprecht R (1998) Marijuana precipitation of panic disorder with agoraphobia. *Acta Psychiatr Scand* 98(3):254–5.

322. Bhattacharyya S, et al. (2014) Impairment of inhibitory control processing related to acute psychotomimetic effects of cannabis. *Eur Neuropsychopharmacol*.

323. Freeman D, et al. (2014) How Cannabis Causes Paranoia: Using the Intravenous Administration of Δ9-Tetrahydrocannabinol (THC) to Identify Key Cognitive Mechanisms Leading to Paranoia. *Schizophr Bull*.

324. Barrowclough C, Gregg L, Lobban F, Bucci S, Emsley R (2014) The Impact of Cannabis Use on Clinical Outcomes in Recent Onset Psychosis. *Schizophr Bull*.

325. Kedzior KK, Laeber LT (2014) A positive association between anxiety disorders and cannabis use or cannabis use disorders in the general population--a meta-analysis of 31 studies. *BMC Psychiatry* 14:136.

326. Hunault CC, et al. (2014) Acute subjective effects after smoking joints containing up to 69 mg Δ9-tetrahydrocannabinol in recreational users: a randomized, crossover clinical trial. *Psychopharmacology (Berl)* 231(24):4723–33.

327. Martin-Santos R, et al. (2012) Acute effects of a single, oral dose of d9-tetrahydrocannabinol (THC) and cannabidiol (CBD) administration in healthy volunteers. *Curr Pharm Des* 18(32):4966–79.

328. Lin H-C, Mao S-C, Chen P-S, Gean P-W (2008) Chronic cannabinoid administration in vivo compromises extinction of fear memory. *Learn Mem* 15(12):876–84.

329. Arendt M, et al. (2007) Testing the self-medication hypothesis of depression and aggression in cannabis-dependent subjects. *Psychol Med* 37(7):935–45.

330. Szuster RR, Pontius EB, Campos PE (1988) Marijuana sensitivity and panic anxiety. *J Clin Psychiatry* 49(11):427–9.

331. Langs G, Fabisch H, Fabisch K, Zapotoczky H (1997) Can cannabis trigger recurrent panic attacks in susceptible patients? *Eur Psychiatry* 12(8):415–9.

332. Patton GC, et al. (2002) Cannabis use and mental health in young people: cohort study. *BMJ* 325(7374):1195–8.

333. Katz G, Durst R, Shufman E, Bar-Hamburger R, Grunhaus L (2010) Cannabis abuse and severity of psychotic and affective disorders in Israeli psychiatric inpatients. *Compr Psychiatry* 51(1):37–41.

334. Marks MA, et al. (2014) Association of marijuana smoking with oropharyngeal and oral tongue cancers: pooled analysis from the INHANCE consortium. *Cancer Epidemiol Biomarkers Prev* 23(1):160–71.

335. Callaghan RC, Allebeck P, Sidorchuk A (2013) Marijuana use and risk of lung cancer: a 40-year cohort study. *Cancer Causes Control* 24(10):1811–20.

336. Hart S, Fischer OM, Ullrich A (2004) Cannabinoids induce cancer cell proliferation via tumor necrosis factor alpha-converting

enzyme (TACE/ADAM17)-mediated transactivation of the epidermal growth factor receptor. *Cancer Res* 64(6):1943–50.

337. Sidney S, Quesenberry CP, Friedman GD, Tekawa IS (1997) Marijuana use and cancer incidence (California, United States). *Cancer Causes Control* 8(5):722–8.

338. Centonze D, et al. (2009) Lack of effect of cannabis-based treatment on clinical and laboratory measures in multiple sclerosis. *Neurol Sci* 30(6):531–4.

339. Lacson JCA, et al. (2012) Population-based case-control study of recreational drug use and testis cancer risk confirms an association between marijuana use and nonseminoma risk. *Cancer* 118(21):5374–83.

340. Kim HR, Son BH, Lee SY, Chung KH, Oh SM (2012) The Role of p53 in Marijuana Smoke Condensates-induced Genotoxicity and Apoptosis. *Environ Health Toxicol* 27:e2012017.

341. Trabert B, Sigurdson AJ, Sweeney AM, Strom SS, McGlynn KA (2011) Marijuana use and testicular germ cell tumors. *Cancer* 117(4):848–53.

342. Zhang ZF, et al. (1999) Marijuana use and increased risk of squamous cell carcinoma of the head and neck. *Cancer Epidemiol Biomarkers Prev* 8(12):1071–8.

343. Daling JR, et al. (2009) Association of marijuana use and the incidence of testicular germ cell tumors. *Cancer* 115(6):1215–23.

344. Pavisian B, et al. (2014) Effects of cannabis on cognition in patients with MS: a psychometric and MRI study. *Neurology* 82(21):1879–87.

345. Honarmand K, Tierney MC, O'Connor P, Feinstein A (2011) Effects of cannabis on cognitive function in patients with multiple sclerosis. *Neurology* 76(13):1153–60.

346. Ghaffar O, Feinstein A (2008) Multiple sclerosis and cannabis: a cognitive and psychiatric study. *Neurology* 71(3):164–9.

347. Rabin RA, Zakzanis KK, Daskalakis ZJ, George TP (2013) Effects of cannabis use status on cognitive function, in males with schizophrenia. *Psychiatry Res* 206(2-3):158–65.

348. Lev-Ran S, et al. (2014) The association between cannabis use and depression: a systematic review and meta-analysis of longitudinal studies. *Psychol Med* 44(4):797–810.

349. Rubino T, et al. (2008) Chronic delta 9-tetrahydrocannabinol during adolescence provokes sex-dependent changes in the emotional profile in adult rats: behavioral and biochemical correlates. *Neuropsychopharmacology* 33(11):2760–71.

350. Cairns KE, Yap MBH, Pilkington PD, Jorm AF (2014) Risk and protective factors for depression that adolescents can modify: a systematic review and meta-analysis of longitudinal studies. *J Affect Disord* 169:61–75.

351. Fairman BJ, Anthony JC (2012) Are early-onset cannabis smokers at an increased risk of depression spells? *J Affect Disord* 138(1-2):54–62.

352. Otten R, Engels RCME (2013) Testing bidirectional effects between cannabis use and depressive symptoms: moderation by the serotonin transporter gene. *Addict Biol* 18(5):826–35.

353. Marmorstein NR, Iacono WG (2011) Explaining associations between cannabis use disorders in adolescence and later major depression: a test of the psychosocial failure model. *Addict Behav* 36(7):773–6.

354. Bovasso GB (2001) Cannabis abuse as a risk factor for depressive symptoms. *Am J Psychiatry* 158(12):2033–7.

355. Ford KA, et al. (2014) Unique functional abnormalities in youth with combined marijuana use and depression: an FMRI study. *Front psychiatry* 5:130.

356. Fergusson DM, Horwood LJ, Swain-Campbell N (2002) Cannabis use and psychosocial adjustment in adolescence and young adulthood. *Addiction* 97(9):1123–35.

357.	Brook DW, Brook JS, Zhang C, Cohen P, Whiteman M (2002) Drug use and the risk of major depressive disorder, alcohol dependence, and substance use disorders. *Arch Gen Psychiatry* 59(11):1039–44.

358.	Nogi M, Fergusson D, Chiaco JMC (2014) Mid-ventricular variant takotsubo cardiomyopathy associated with Cannabinoid Hyperemesis Syndrome: a case report. *Hawaii J Med Public Health* 73(4):115–8.

359.	Vaziri ND, et al. (1981) Toxicity with intravenous injection of crude marijuana extract. *Clin Toxicol* 18(3):353–66.

360.	Nicolson SE, Denysenko L, Mulcare JL, Vito JP, Chabon B ' Cannabinoid hyperemesis syndrome: a case series and review of previous reports. *Psychosomatics* 53(3):212–9.

361.	Simonetto DA, Oxentenko AS, Herman ML, Szostek JH (2012) Cannabinoid hyperemesis: a case series of 98 patients. *Mayo Clin Proc* 87(2):114–9.

362.	Allen JH, de Moore GM, Heddle R, Twartz JC (2004) Cannabinoid hyperemesis: cyclical hyperemesis in association with chronic cannabis abuse. *Gut* 53(11):1566–70.

363.	Muschart X, Flament J (2015) A non-classical cannabinoid syndrome. *Acta Clin Belg*:2295333714Y0000000116.

364.	Hézode C, et al. (2005) Daily cannabis smoking as a risk factor for progression of fibrosis in chronic hepatitis C. *Hepatology* 42(1):63–71.

365.	Hézode C, et al. (2008) Daily cannabis use: a novel risk factor of steatosis severity in patients with chronic hepatitis C. *Gastroenterology* 134(2):432–9.

366.	Ishida JH, et al. (2008) Influence of cannabis use on severity of hepatitis C disease. *Clin Gastroenterol Hepatol* 6(1):69–75.

367.	Mallat A, Hezode C, Lotersztajn S (2008) Environmental factors as disease accelerators during chronic hepatitis C. *J Hepatol* 48(4):657–65.

368. Borini P, Guimarães RC, Borini SB (2004) Possible hepatotoxicity of chronic marijuana usage. *Sao Paulo Med J* 122(3):110–6.

369. Clark WC, Janal MN, Zeidenberg P, Nahas GG (1981) Effects of moderate and high doses of marihuana on thermal pain: a sensory decision theory analysis. *J Clin Pharmacol* 21(8-9 Suppl):299S–310S.

370. Benowitz NL, Rosenberg J, Rogers W, Bachman J, Jones RT (1979) Cardiovascular effects of intravenous delta-9-tetrahydrocannabinol: autonomic nervous mechanisms. *Clin Pharmacol Ther* 25(4):440–6.

371. Cabral GA, Pettit DA, Fischer-Stenger K (1993) Marijuana and host resistance to herpesvirus infection. *Adv Exp Med Biol* 335:95–106.

372. Fischer-Stenger K, Updegrove AW, Cabral GA (1992) Delta 9-tetrahydrocannabinol decreases cytotoxic T lymphocyte activity to herpes simplex virus type 1-infected cells. *Proc Soc Exp Biol Med* 200(3):422–30.

373. Specter S, Lancz G, Westrich G, Friedman H (1991) Delta-9-tetrahydrocannabinol augments murine retroviral induced immunosuppression and infection. *Int J Immunopharmacol* 13(4):411–7.

374. Morahan PS, Klykken PC, Smith SH, Harris LS, Munson AE (1979) Effects of cannabinoids on host resistance to Listeria monocytogenes and herpes simplex virus. *Infect Immun* 23(3):670–4.

375. Killestein J, et al. (2002) Safety, tolerability, and efficacy of orally administered cannabinoids in MS. *Neurology* 58(9):1404–7.

376. Greenberg HS, et al. (1994) Short-term effects of smoking marijuana on balance in patients with multiple sclerosis and normal volunteers. *Clin Pharmacol Ther* 55(3):324–8.

377. Rais M, et al. (2008) Excessive brain volume loss over time in cannabis-using first-episode schizophrenia patients. *Am J Psychiatry* 165(4):490–6.

378. Zhornitsky S, et al. (2010) Extrapyramidal symptoms in substance abusers with and without schizophrenia and in nonabusing patients with schizophrenia. *Mov Disord* 25(13):2188–94.

379. Welch KA, et al. (2011) The impact of substance use on brain structure in people at high risk of developing schizophrenia. *Schizophr Bull* 37(5):1066–76.

380. Wobrock T, et al. (2010) Increased cortical inhibition deficits in first-episode schizophrenia with comorbid cannabis abuse. *Psychopharmacology (Berl)* 208(3):353–63.

381. Bhattacharyya S, et al. (2009) Modulation of mediotemporal and ventrostriatal function in humans by Delta9-tetrahydrocannabinol: a neural basis for the effects of Cannabis sativa on learning and psychosis. *Arch Gen Psychiatry* 66(4):442–51.

382. Rentzsch J, et al. (2007) Differential impact of heavy cannabis use on sensory gating in schizophrenic patients and otherwise healthy controls. *Exp Neurol* 205(1):241–9.

383. Szeszko PR, et al. (2007) Anterior cingulate grey-matter deficits and cannabis use in first-episode schizophrenia. *Br J Psychiatry* 190:230–6.

384. Skosnik PD, Krishnan GP, Aydt EE, Kuhlenshmidt HA, O'Donnell BF (2006) Psychophysiological evidence of altered neural synchronization in cannabis use: relationship to schizotypy. *Am J Psychiatry* 163(10):1798–805.

385. Kedzior KK, Martin-Iverson MT (2006) Chronic cannabis use is associated with attention-modulated reduction in prepulse inhibition of the startle reflex in healthy humans. *J Psychopharmacol* 20(4):471–84.

386. Jockers-Scherübl MC, et al. (2004) Brain-derived neurotrophic factor serum concentrations are increased in drug-naive schizophrenic patients with chronic cannabis abuse and multiple substance abuse. *Neurosci Lett* 371(1):79–83.

387. Epstein KA, Kumra S (2015) Altered cortical maturation in adolescent cannabis users with and without schizophrenia. *Schizophr Res*.

388. Kvitland LR, et al. (2014) Cannabis use in first-treatment bipolar I disorder: relations to clinical characteristics. *Early Interv Psychiatry*.

389. Zorrilla I, et al. (2014) Cannabis and bipolar disorder: does quitting cannabis use during manic/mixed episode improve clinical/functional outcomes? *Acta Psychiatr Scand*.

390. Gibbs M, et al. (2014) Cannabis use and mania symptoms: A systematic review and meta-analysis. *J Affect Disord* 171C:39–47.

391. Khan MA, Akella S (2009) Cannabis-induced bipolar disorder with psychotic features: a case report. *Psychiatry (Edgmont)* 6(12):44–8.

392. Van Rossum I, Boomsma M, Tenback D, Reed C, van Os J (2009) Does cannabis use affect treatment outcome in bipolar disorder? A longitudinal analysis. *J Nerv Ment Dis* 197(1):35–40.

393. Baethge C, et al. (2008) Sequencing of substance use and affective morbidity in 166 first-episode bipolar I disorder patients. *Bipolar Disord* 10(6):738–41.

394. Goldberg JF, Garno JL, Leon AC, Kocsis JH, Portera L (1999) A history of substance abuse complicates remission from acute mania in bipolar disorder. *J Clin Psychiatry* 60(11):733–40.

395. Kibby T, Halcomb SE (2013) Toxicology observation: nystagmus after marijuana use. *J Forensic Leg Med* 20(4):345–6.

396. Aharonovich E, et al. (2005) Postdischarge cannabis use and its relationship to cocaine, alcohol, and heroin use: a prospective study. *Am J Psychiatry* 162(8):1507–14.

397. Hermann D, Klages E, Welzel H, Mann K, Croissant B (2005) Low efficacy of non-opioid drugs in opioid withdrawal symptoms. *Addict Biol* 10(2):165–9.

398. Wasserman DA, Weinstein MG, Havassy BE, Hall SM (1998) Factors associated with lapses to heroin use during methadone maintenance. *Drug Alcohol Depend* 52(3):183–92.

399. Mikolašević I, Milić S, Mijandrušić-Sinčić B, Licul V, Štimac D (2013) Cannabis-induced acute pancreatitis. *Med Glas (Zenica)* 10(2):405–7.

400. Howaizi M, Chahine M, Haydar F, Jemaa Y, Lapoile E (2012) Cannabis-induced recurrent acute pancreatitis. *Acta Gastroenterol Belg* 75(4):446–7.

401. Fatma H, Mouna B, Leila M, Radhouane D, Taoufik N (2013) Cannabis: a rare cause of acute pancreatitis. *Clin Res Hepatol Gastroenterol* 37(1):e24–5.

402. Wargo KA, Geveden BN, McConnell VJ (2007) Cannabinoid-induced pancreatitis: a case series. *JOP* 8(5):579–83.

403. Grant P, Gandhi P (2004) A case of cannabis-induced pancreatitis. *JOP* 5(1):41–3.

404. Fogang YF, Camara M, Mbonda PC, Toffa D, Touré K (2014) Late onset epilepsy associated with marijuana abuse: a case report with MRI findings. *Pan Afr Med J* 17:158.

405. Trojak B, et al. (2011) Stroke with neuropsychiatric sequelae after cannabis use in a man: a case report. *J Med Case Rep* 5:264.

406. Bonkowsky JL, Sarco D, Pomeroy SL (2005) Ataxia and shaking in a 2-year-old girl: acute marijuana intoxication presenting as seizure. *Pediatr Emerg Care* 21(8):527–8.

407. Consroe P, Fish BS (1981) Rabbit behavioral model of marijuana psychoactivity in humans. *Med Hypotheses* 7(8):1079–90.

408. Martin P, Consroe P (1976) Cannabinoid induced behavioral convulsions in rabbits. *Science* 194(4268):965–7.

409. Camera AA, et al. (2012) Correlates to the variable effects of cannabis in young adults: a preliminary study. *Harm Reduct J* 9:15.

410. Degenhardt L, et al. (2007) The temporal dynamics of relationships between cannabis, psychosis and depression among young adults with psychotic disorders: findings from a 10-month prospective study. *Psychol Med* 37(7):927–34.

411. Van Gastel WA, et al. (2014) Change in cannabis use in the general population: a longitudinal study on the impact on psychotic experiences. *Schizophr Res* 157(1-3):266–70.

412. Peters BD, et al. (2009) Subjective effects of cannabis before the first psychotic episode. *Aust N Z J Psychiatry* 43(12):1155–62.

413. Torrey EF, Bartko JJ, Yolken RH (2012) Toxoplasma gondii and other risk factors for schizophrenia: an update. *Schizophr Bull* 38(3):642–7.

414. Corcoran CM, et al. (2008) Temporal association of cannabis use with symptoms in individuals at clinical high risk for psychosis. *Schizophr Res* 106(2-3):286–93.

415. D'Souza DC, et al. (2004) The psychotomimetic effects of intravenous delta-9-tetrahydrocannabinol in healthy individuals: implications for psychosis. *Neuropsychopharmacology* 29(8):1558–72.

416. Foti DJ, Kotov R, Guey LT, Bromet EJ (2010) Cannabis use and the course of schizophrenia: 10-year follow-up after first hospitalization. *Am J Psychiatry* 167(8):987–93.

417. Skinner R, Conlon L, Gibbons D, McDonald C (2011) Cannabis use and non-clinical dimensions of psychosis in university students presenting to primary care. *Acta Psychiatr Scand* 123(1):21–7.

418. Hides L, Dawe S, Kavanagh DJ, Young RM (2006) Psychotic symptom and cannabis relapse in recent-onset psychosis. Prospective study. *Br J Psychiatry* 189:137–43.

419. Hides L, et al. (2009) The association between early cannabis use and psychotic-like experiences in a community adolescent sample. *Schizophr Res* 112(1-3):130–5.

420. Kulhalli V, Isaac M, Murthy P (2007) Cannabis-related psychosis: Presentation and effect of abstinence. *Indian J Psychiatry* 49(4):256–61.

421. Scherr M, et al. (2012) Environmental risk factors and their impact on the age of onset of schizophrenia: Comparing familial to non-familial schizophrenia. *Nord J Psychiatry* 66(2):107–14.

422. Fridberg DJ, Vollmer JM, O'Donnell BF, Skosnik PD (2011) Cannabis users differ from non-users on measures of personality and schizotypy. *Psychiatry Res* 186(1):46–52.

423. Batki SL, Leontieva L, Dimmock JA, Ploutz-Snyder R (2008) Negative symptoms are associated with less alcohol use, craving, and "high" in alcohol dependent patients with schizophrenia. *Schizophr Res* 105(1-3):201–7.

424. Bahorik AL, et al. (2014) BRIEF REPORT: THE IMPACT OF ALCOHOL AND CANNABIS MISUSE ON COGNITION AMONG INDIVIDUALS WITH SCHIZOPHRENIA. *Schizophr Res Cogn* 1(3):160–163.

425. Manrique-Garcia E, et al. (2014) Prognosis of schizophrenia in persons with and without a history of cannabis use. *Psychol Med* 44(12):2513–21.

426. Stefanis NC, et al. (2013) Age at initiation of cannabis use predicts age at onset of psychosis: the 7- to 8-year trend. *Schizophr Bull* 39(2):251–4.

427. Stefanis NC, et al. (2014) The effect of drug use on the age at onset of psychotic disorders in an Australian cohort. *Schizophr Res* 156(2-3):211–6.

428. Davis GP, Compton MT, Wang S, Levin FR, Blanco C (2013) Association between cannabis use, psychosis, and schizotypal personality disorder: findings from the National Epidemiologic Survey on Alcohol and Related Conditions. *Schizophr Res* 151(1-3):197–202.

429. Stone JM, et al. (2014) Cannabis use and first-episode psychosis: relationship with manic and psychotic symptoms, and with age at presentation. *Psychol Med* 44(3):499–506.

430. Clausen L, et al. (2014) Change in cannabis use, clinical symptoms and social functioning among patients with first-episode psychosis: a 5-year follow-up study of patients in the OPUS trial. *Psychol Med* 44(1):117–26.

431. Niemi-Pynttäri JA, et al. (2013) Substance-induced psychoses converting into schizophrenia: a register-based study of 18,478 Finnish inpatient cases. *J Clin Psychiatry* 74(1):e94–9.

432. Power BD, Dragovic M, Jablensky A, Stefanis NC (2013) Does accumulating exposure to illicit drugs bring forward the age at onset in schizophrenia? *Aust N Z J Psychiatry* 47(1):51–8.

433. Ringen PA, et al. (2013) Cannabis use and premorbid functioning as predictors of poorer neurocognition in schizophrenia spectrum disorder. *Schizophr Res* 143(1):84–9.

434. Khan MK, Usmani MA, Hanif SA (2012) A case of self amputa-tion of penis by cannabis induced psychosis. *J Forensic Leg Med* 19(6):355–7.

435. Galvez-Buccollini JA, et al. (2012) Association between age at onset of psychosis and age at onset of cannabis use in non-affec-tive psychosis. *Schizophr Res* 139(1-3):157–60.

436. Myles N, Newall H, Nielssen O, Large M (2012) The association between cannabis use and earlier age at onset of schizophrenia and other psychoses: meta-analysis of possible confounding fac-tors. *Curr Pharm Des* 18(32):5055–69.

437. Husted JA, Ahmed R, Chow EWC, Brzustowicz LM, Bassett AS (2012) Early environmental exposures influence schizophrenia expression even in the presence of strong genetic predisposition. *Schizophr Res* 137(1-3):166–8.

438. Rössler W, Hengartner MP, Angst J, Ajdacic-Gross V (2012) Linking substance use with symptoms of subclinical psychosis in a com-munity cohort over 30 years. *Addiction* 107(6):1174–84.

439. Dragt S, et al. (2012) Cannabis use and age at onset of symptoms in subjects at clinical high risk for psychosis. *Acta Psychiatr Scand* 125(1):45–53.

440. Dragt S, et al. (2010) Age of onset of cannabis use is associated with age of onset of high-risk symptoms for psychosis. *Can J Psychiatry* 55(3):165–71.

441. Harley M, et al. (2010) Cannabis use and childhood trauma inter-act additively to increase the risk of psychotic symptoms in ado-lescence. *Psychol Med* 40(10):1627–34.

442. Compton MT, Chien VH, Bollini AM (2009) Associations between past alcohol, cannabis, and cocaine use and current schizotypy among first-degree relatives of patients with schizophrenia and non-psychiatric controls. *Psychiatr Q* 80(3):143–54.

443. Compton MT, et al. (2009) Association of pre-onset cannabis, alcohol, and tobacco use with age at onset of prodrome and age

at onset of psychosis in first-episode patients. *Am J Psychiatry* 166(11):1251–7.

444. Sugranyes G, et al. (2009) Cannabis use and age of diagnosis of schizophrenia. *Eur Psychiatry* 24(5):282–6.

445. Barkus EJ, Stirling J, Hopkins RS, Lewis S (2006) Cannabis-induced psychosis-like experiences are associated with high schizotypy. *Psychopathology* 39(4):175–8.

446. Rehman IU, Farooq S (2007) Schizophrenia and comorbid self reported cannabis abuse: impact on course, functioning and services use. *J Pak Med Assoc* 57(2):60–4.

447. Rössler W, et al. (2007) Psychotic experiences in the general population: a twenty-year prospective community study. *Schizophr Res* 92(1-3):1–14.

448. Barnes TRE, Mutsatsa SH, Hutton SB, Watt HC, Joyce EM (2006) Comorbid substance use and age at onset of schizophrenia. *Br J Psychiatry* 188:237–42.

449. Grech A, Van Os J, Jones PB, Lewis SW, Murray RM (2005) Cannabis use and outcome of recent onset psychosis. *Eur Psychiatry* 20(4):349–53.

450. Henquet C, Murray R, Linszen D, van Os J (2005) The environment and schizophrenia: the role of cannabis use. *Schizophr Bull* 31(3):608–12.

451. Semple DM, McIntosh AM, Lawrie SM (2005) Cannabis as a risk factor for psychosis: systematic review. *J Psychopharmacol* 19(2):187–94.

452. Isaac M, Isaac M, Holloway F (2005) Is cannabis an anti-anti-psychotic? The experience in psychiatric intensive care. *Hum Psychopharmacol* 20(3):207–10.

453. Veen ND, et al. (2004) Cannabis use and age at onset of schizophrenia. *Am J Psychiatry* 161(3):501–6.

454. Degenhardt L, Hall W, Lynskey M (2003) Testing hypotheses about the relationship between cannabis use and psychosis. *Drug Alcohol Depend* 71(1):37–48.

455. Arseneault L, et al. (2002) Cannabis use in adolescence and risk for adult psychosis: longitudinal prospective study. *BMJ* 325(7374):1212–3.

456. Zammit S, Allebeck P, Andreasson S, Lundberg I, Lewis G (2002) Self reported cannabis use as a risk factor for schizophrenia in Swedish conscripts of 1969: historical cohort study. *BMJ* 325(7374):1199.

457. Caspari D (1999) Cannabis and schizophrenia: results of a follow-up study. *Eur Arch Psychiatry Clin Neurosci* 249(1):45–9.

458. Baigent M, Holme G, Hafner RJ (1995) Self reports of the interaction between substance abuse and schizophrenia. *Aust N Z J Psychiatry* 29(1):69–74.

459. Linszen DH, Dingemans PM, Lenior ME (1994) Cannabis abuse and the course of recent-onset schizophrenic disorders. *Arch Gen Psychiatry* 51(4):273–9.

460. Andréasson S, Allebeck P, Engström A, Rydberg U (1987) Cannabis and schizophrenia. A longitudinal study of Swedish conscripts. *Lancet* 2(8574):1483–6.

461. Andréasson S, Allebeck P, Rydberg U (1989) Schizophrenia in users and nonusers of cannabis. A longitudinal study in Stockholm County. *Acta Psychiatr Scand* 79(5):505–10.

462. Negrete JC, Knapp WP, Douglas DE, Smith WB (1986) Cannabis affects the severity of schizophrenic symptoms: results of a clinical survey. *Psychol Med* 16(3):515–20.

463. Day NL, Goldschmidt L, Day R, Larkby C, Richardson GA (2014) Prenatal marijuana exposure, age of marijuana initiation, and the development of psychotic symptoms in young adults. *Psychol Med*:1–9.

464. Moore BA, Augustson EM, Moser RP, Budney AJ (2005) Respiratory effects of marijuana and tobacco use in a U.S. sample. *J Gen Intern Med* 20(1):33–7.

465. Vidal C, Fuente R, Iglesias A, Sáez A (1991) Bronchial asthma due to Cannabis sativa seed. *Allergy* 46(8):647–9.

466. Tashkin DP, Simmons MS, Tseng C-H (2012) Impact of changes in regular use of marijuana and/or tobacco on chronic bronchitis. *COPD* 9(4):367–74.

467. Beshay M, Kaiser H, Niedhart D, Reymond MA, Schmid RA (2007) Emphysema and secondary pneumothorax in young adults smoking cannabis. *Eur J Cardiothorac Surg* 32(6):834–8.

468. Sherrill DL, Krzyzanowski M, Bloom JW, Lebowitz MD (1991) Respiratory effects of non-tobacco cigarettes: a longitudinal study in general population. *Int J Epidemiol* 20(1):132–7.

469. Morris RR (1985) Human pulmonary histopathological changes from marijuana smoking. *J Forensic Sci* 30(2):345–9.

470. Gao Z, et al. (2010) "Bong lung" in cystic fibrosis: a case report. *J Med Case Rep* 4:371.

471. Malit LA, et al. (1975) Intravenous delta9-Tetrahydrocannabinol: Effects of ventilatory control and cardiovascular dynamics. *Anesthesiology* 42(6):666–73.

472. Robert T, Kawkabani Marchini A, Oumarou G, Uské A (2013) Reversible cerebral vasoconstriction syndrome identification of prognostic factors. *Clin Neurol Neurosurg* 115(11):2351–7.

473. Ngaotepprutaram T, Kaplan BLF, Crawford RB, Kaminski NE (2012) Differential modulation by delta9-tetrahydrocannabinol (Δ9)-THC) of CD40 ligand (CD40L) expression in activated mouse splenic CD4+ T cells. *J Neuroimmune Pharmacol* 7(4):969–80.

474. Haney M, et al. (2007) Dronabinol and marijuana in HIV-positive marijuana smokers. Caloric intake, mood, and sleep. *J Acquir Immune Defic Syndr* 45(5):545–554.

475. James J (2000) Marijuana safety study completed: weight gain, no safety problems. *AIDS Treat News* Aug 4(348):3–4.

476. Aragona M, et al. (2009) Psychopathological and cognitive effects of therapeutic cannabinoids in multiple sclerosis: a double-blind, placebo controlled, crossover study. *Clin Neuropharmacol* 32(1):41–7.

477. Sidney S (2001) Marijuana use in HIV-positive and AIDS patients: Results of a an anonymous mail survey. *J Cannabis Ther* 1(3-4):35–43.

478. Ogborne AC, Smart RG, Weber T, Birchmore-Timney C (2000) Who is using cannabis as a medicine and why: an exploratory study. *J Psychoactive Drugs* 32(4):435–43.

479. Lutge EE, Gray A, Siegfried N (2013) The medical use of cannabis for reducing morbidity and mortality in patients with HIV/AIDS. *Cochrane database Syst Rev* 4:CD005175.

480. Abrams DI, et al. (2003) Short-term effects of cannabinoids in patients with HIV-1 infection: a randomized, placebo-controlled clinical trial. *Ann Intern Med* 139(4):258–66.

481. Zumbrun EE, Sido JM, Nagarkatti PS, Nagarkatti M (2015) Epigenetic Regulation of Immunological Alterations Following Prenatal Exposure to Marijuana Cannabinoids and its Long Term Consequences in Offspring. *J Neuroimmune Pharmacol*.

482. Aso E, Sanchez-Pla A, Vegas-Lozano E, Maldonado R, Ferrer I (2015) Cannabis-Based Medicine Reduces Multiple Pathological Processes in AβPP/PS1 Mice. *J Alzheimers Dis* 43(3):977–991.

483. Volicer L, Stelly M, Morris J, McLaughlin J, Volicer BJ (1997) Effects of dronabinol on anorexia and disturbed behavior in patients with Alzheimer's disease. *Int J Geriatr Psychiatry* 12(9):913–9.

484. Cao C, et al. (2014) The potential therapeutic effects of THC on Alzheimer's disease. *J Alzheimers Dis* 42(3):973–84.

485. Carter G, Abood M, Aggarwal S, Weiss M (2010) Cannabis and amyotrophic lateral sclerosis: hypothetical and practical applications and a call for clinical trials. *Am J Hosp Palliat Care* 27(5):347–356.

486. Weydt P, et al. (2005) Cannabinol delays symptom onset in SOD1 (G93A) transgenic mice without affecting survival. *Amyotroph Lateral Scler Other Mot Neuron Disord* 6(3):182–184.

487. Carter G, Rosen B (2001) Marijuana in the management of amyotrophic lateral sclerosis. *Am J Hosp Palliat Care* 18:264–270.

488. Moreno-Martet M, Espejo-Porras F, Fernández-Ruiz J, de Lago E (2014) Changes in endocannabinoid receptors and enzymes in the spinal cord of SOD1(G93A) transgenic mice and evaluation of a Sativex(®) -like combination of phytocannabinoids: interest for future therapies in amyotrophic lateral sclerosis. *CNS Neurosci Ther* 20(9):809–15.

489. Costiniuk CT, Mills E, Cooper CL (2008) Evaluation of oral cannabinoid-containing medications for the management of interferon and ribavirin-induced anorexia, nausea and weight loss in patients treated for chronic hepatitis C virus. *Can J Gastroenterol* 22(4):376–80.

490. Naftali T, Mechulam R, Lev LB, Konikoff FM (2014) Cannabis for inflammatory bowel disease. *Dig Dis* 32(4):468–74.

491. Consroe P, Musty R, Rein J, Tillery W, Pertwee R (1997) The perceived effects of smoked cannabis on patients with multiple sclerosis. *Eur Neurol* 38(1):44–8.

492. Morgan C, Freeman T, Schafer G, Curran H (2010) Cannabidiol attenuates the appetitive effects of Delta 9-tetrahydrocannabinol in humans smoking their chosen cannabis. *Neuropsychopharmacology* 35(9):1879–1885.

493. Woolridge E, et al. (2005) Cannabis use in HIV for pain and other medical symptoms. *J Pain Symptom Manage* 29(4):358–67.

494. Sofia RD, Knobloch LC (1976) Comparative effects of various naturally occurring cannabinoids on food, sucrose and water consumption by rats. *Pharmacol Biochem Behav* 4(5):591–9.

495. Fukuda S, et al. (2014) Cannabinoid receptor 2 as a potential therapeutic target in rheumatoid arthritis. *BMC Musculoskelet Disord* 15:275.

496. Jeong M, et al. (2014) Hempseed oil induces reactive oxygen species- and C/EBP homologous protein-mediated apoptosis in MH7A human rheumatoid arthritis fibroblast-like synovial cells. *J Ethnopharmacol* 154(3):745–52.

497. Richardson D, et al. (2008) Characterisation of the cannabinoid receptor system in synovial tissue and fluid in patients with osteoarthritis and rheumatoid arthritis. *Arthritis Res Ther* 10(2):R43.

498. George KL, Saltman LH, Stein GS, Lian JB, Zurier RB (2008) Ajulemic acid, a nonpsychoactive cannabinoid acid, suppresses osteoclastogenesis in mononuclear precursor cells and induces apoptosis in mature osteoclast-like cells. *J Cell Physiol* 214(3):714–20.

499. Zurier RB, Rossetti RG, Burstein SH, Bidinger B (2003) Suppression of human monocyte interleukin-1beta production by ajulemic acid, a nonpsychoactive cannabinoid. *Biochem Pharmacol* 65(4):649–55.

500. Russo E, Guy GW (2006) A tale of two cannabinoids: the therapeutic rationale for combining tetrahydrocannabinol and cannabidiol. *Med Hypotheses* 66(2):234–46.

501. Brophy S, Calin A (2002) Definition of disease flare in ankylosing spondylitis: the patients' perspective. *J Rheumatol* 29(5):954–8.

502. Husni AS, et al. (2014) Evaluation of Phytocannabinoids from High Potency Cannabis sativa using In Vitro Bioassays to Determine Structure-Activity Relationships for Cannabinoid Receptor 1 and Cannabinoid Receptor 2. *Med Chem Res* 23(9):4295–4300.

503. Takeda S, et al. (2014) Δ(9)-THC modulation of fatty acid 2-hydroxylase (FA2H) gene expression: Possible involvement of induced levels of PPARα in MDA-MB-231 breast cancer cells. *Toxicology* 326:18–24.

504. Bar-Sela G, et al. (2013) The medical necessity for medicinal cannabis: prospective, observational study evaluating the treatment in cancer patients on supportive or palliative care. *Evid Based Complement Alternat Med* 2013:510392.

505. De Petrocellis L, et al. (2011) Effects of cannabinoids and cannabinoid-enriched Cannabis extracts on TRP channels and endocannabinoid metabolic enzymes. *Br J Pharmacol* 163(7):1479–94.

506. Waissengrin B, Urban D, Leshem Y, Garty M, Wolf I (2014) Patterns of Use of Medical Cannabis Among Israeli Cancer Patients: A Single Institution Experience. *J Pain Symptom Manage.*

507.   Liang C, et al. (2009) A population-based case-control study of marijuana use and head and neck squamous cell carcinoma. *Cancer Prev Res* 2(8):759–768.

508.   Hong Y, et al. (2013) PPARγ mediates the effects of WIN55,212-2, an synthetic cannabinoid, on the proliferation and apoptosis of the BEL-7402 hepatocarcinoma cells. *Mol Biol Rep* 40(11):6287–93.

509.   Salazar M, et al. (2013) The pseudokinase tribbles homologue-3 plays a crucial role in cannabinoid anticancer action. *Biochim Biophys Acta* 1831(10):1573–8.

510.   Moreno E, et al. (2014) Targeting CB2-GPR55 receptor heteromers modulates cancer cell signaling. *J Biol Chem* 289(32):21960–72.

511.   Sánchez C, Galve-Roperh I, Canova C, Brachet P, Guzmán M (1998) Delta9-tetrahydrocannabinol induces apoptosis in C6 glioma cells. *FEBS Lett* 436(1):6–10.

512.   Thomas AA, et al. (2015) Association Between Cannabis Use and the Risk of Bladder Cancer: Results From the California Men's Health Study. *Urology* 85(2):388–93.

513.   Berthiller J, et al. (2009) Marijuana smoking and the risk of head and neck cancer: pooled analysis in the INHANCE consortium. *Cancer Epidemiol Biomarkers Prev* 18(5):1544–51.

514.   Aldington S, et al. (2008) Cannabis use and cancer of the head and neck: case-control study. *Otolaryngol Head Neck Surg* 138(3):374–80.

515.   Hashibe M, et al. (2006) Marijuana use and the risk of lung and upper aerodigestive tract cancers: results of a population-based case-control study. *Cancer Epidemiol Biomarkers Prev* 15(10):1829–34.

516.   Hollister L (1971) Hunger and appetite after single doses of marihuana, alcohol, and dextroamphetamine. *Clin Pharmacol Ther* 12:44–49.

517.   Abel E (1971) Effects of marihuana on the solution of anagrams, memory and appetite. *Nature* 231:260–261.

518. Jamshidi N, Taylor DA (2001) Anandamide administration into the ventromedial hypothalamus stimulates appetite in rats. *Br J Pharmacol* 134(6):1151–4.

519. Lim MP, Devi LA, Rozenfeld R (2011) Cannabidiol causes activated hepatic stellate cell death through a mechanism of endoplasmic reticulum stress-induced apoptosis. *Cell Death Dis* 2:e170.

520. Brunet L, et al. (2013) Marijuana smoking does not accelerate progression of liver disease in HIV-hepatitis C coinfection: a longitudinal cohort analysis. *Clin Infect Dis* 57(5):663–70.

521. Naftali T, et al. (2011) Treatment of Crohn's disease with cannabis: an observational study. *Isr Med Assoc J* 13(8):455–8.

522. Schicho R, Storr M (2014) Cannabis finds its way into treatment of Crohn's disease. *Pharmacology* 93(1-2):1–3.

523. Lal S, et al. (2011) Cannabis use amongst patients with inflammatory bowel disease. *Eur J Gastroenterol Hepatol* 23(10):891–6.

524. Snider S, Consroe P (1984) Treatment of Meige's syndrome with cannabidiol. *Neurology* 34(Suppl):147.

525. Sandyk R, Snider S, Consroe P, Elias S (1986) Cannabidiol in dystonic movement disorders. *Psychiatry Res* 18:291.

526. Chatterjee A, Almahrezi A, Ware M, Fitzcharles M-A (2002) A dramatic response to inhaled cannabis in a woman with central thalamic pain and dystonia. *J Pain Symptom Manage* 24(1):4–6.

527. Lorenz R (2004) On the application of cannabis in paediatrics and epileptology. *Neuro Endocrinol Lett* 25(1-2):40–4.

528. Brust J, Ng S, Hauser A, Susser M (1992) Marijuana use and the risk of new onset seizures. *Trans Am Clin Climatol Assoc* 103:176–181.

529. Zhornitsky S, Potvin S (2012) Cannabidiol in humans-the quest for therapeutic targets. *Pharmaceuticals (Basel)* 5(5):529–52.

530. Ladino LD, Hernández-Ronquillo L, Téllez-Zenteno JF (2014) Medicinal marijuana for epilepsy: a case series study. *Can J Neurol Sci* 41(6):753–8.

531.   McConnell B V, Applegate M, Keniston A, Kluger B, Maa EH (2014)
       Use of complementary and alternative medicine in an urban
       county hospital epilepsy clinic. *Epilepsy Behav* 34:73–6.

532.   Porter BE, Jacobson C (2013) Report of a parent survey of can-
       nabidiol-enriched cannabis use in pediatric treatment-resistant
       epilepsy. *Epilepsy Behav* 29(3):574–7.

533.   Hill KP, et al. (2013) Association of cannabis use with opioid out-
       comes among opioid-dependent youth. *Drug Alcohol Depend*
       132(1-2):342–5.

534.   Corral V (2001) Differential effects of medical marijuana based
       on strain and route of administration: A three-year observational
       study. *J cannabis Ther* 1(3-4):43–59.

535.   Hamerle M, Ghaeni L, Kowski A, Weissinger F, Holtkamp M (2014)
       Cannabis and other illicit drug use in epilepsy patients. *Eur J Neurol*
       21(1):167–70.

536.   Schley M, et al. (2006) Delta-9-THC based monotherapy in fibro-
       myalgia patients on experimentally induced pain, axon reflex
       flare, and pain relief. *Curr Med Res Opin* 22(7):1269–76.

537.   Flach AJ (2002) Delta-9-tetrahydrocannabinol (THC) in the treat-
       ment of end-stage open-angle glaucoma. *Trans Am Ophthalmol
       Soc* 100:215–22; discussion 222–4.

538.   Porcella A, Maxia C, Gessa GL, Pani L (2000) The human eye
       expresses high levels of CB1 cannabinoid receptor mRNA and
       protein. *Eur J Neurosci* 12(3):1123–7.

539.   Porcella A, Casellas P, Gessa GL, Pani L (1998) Cannabinoid recep-
       tor CB1 mRNA is highly expressed in the rat ciliary body: implica-
       tions for the antiglaucoma properties of marihuana. *Brain Res Mol
       Brain Res* 58(1-2):240–5.

540.   Porcella A, Maxia C, Gessa GL, Pani L (2001) The synthetic canna-
       binoid WIN55212-2 decreases the intraocular pressure in human
       glaucoma resistant to conventional therapies. *Eur J Neurosci*
       13(2):409–12.

541. Merritt JC, Olsen JL, Armstrong JR, McKinnon SM (1981) Topical delta 9-tetrahydrocannabinol in hypertensive glaucomas. *J Pharm Pharmacol* 33(1):40–1.

542. Merritt JC, Perry DD, Russell DN, Jones BF (1981) Topical delta 9-tetrahydrocannabinol and aqueous dynamics in glaucoma. *J Clin Pharmacol* 21(8-9 Suppl):467S–471S.

543. Perez-Reyes M, WAgner D, Wall M, Davis K (1976) Intravenous administration of cannabinoids and intraocular pressure. *Pharmacoogy of Marihuana*, eds Braude M, Szara S (Raven Press, New York), pp 829–832.

544. Hepler R, Frank I (1971) Marihuana smoking and intraocular pressure. *J Am Med Assoc* 217:1392.

545. Hepler R, Frank I, Petrus R (1976) Ocular effects of marijuana smoking. *The Pharmacology of Marihuana*, eds Braude M, Szara S (Raven Press, New York), pp 815–828.

546. Deutsch HM, Green K, Zalkow LH (1981) Isolation of ocular hypotensive agents from Cannabis sativa. *J Clin Pharmacol* 21(8-9 Suppl):479S–485S.

547. Sylvestre DL, Clements BJ, Malibu Y (2006) Cannabis use improves retention and virological outcomes in patients treated for hepatitis C. *Eur J Gastroenterol Hepatol* 18(10):1057–63.

548. Liu T, et al. (2014) Marijuana use in hepatitis C infection does not affect liver biopsy histology or treatment outcomes. *Can J Gastroenterol Hepatol* 28(7):381–4.

549. Russell M, et al. (2014) The impact of lifetime drug use on hepatitis C treatment outcomes in insured members of an integrated health care plan. *Drug Alcohol Depend* 134:222–7.

550. Uritsky TJ, McPherson ML, Pradel F (2011) Assessment of hospice health professionals' knowledge, views, and experience with medical marijuana. *J Palliat Med* 14(12):1291–5.

551. Carter GT, et al. (2011) Cannabis in palliative medicine: improving care and reducing opioid-related morbidity. *Am J Hosp Palliat Care* 28(5):297–303.

552. Klumpers LE, et al. (2012) Novel Δ(9) -tetrahydrocannabinol for-
      mulation Namisol® has beneficial pharmacokinetics and promis-
      ing pharmacodynamic effects. *Br J Clin Pharmacol* 74(1):42–53.

553. Chiarlone A, et al. (2014) A restricted population of CB1 cannabi-
      noid receptors with neuroprotective activity. *Proc Natl Acad Sci U S
      A* 111(22):8257–62.

554. Meisel K, Friedman JH (2012) Medical marijuana in Huntington's
      disease: report of two cases. *Med Health R I* 95(6):178–9.

555. Valdeolivas S, Satta V, Pertwee RG, Fernández-Ruiz J, Sagredo O
      (2012) Sativex-like combination of phytocannabinoids is neuro-
      protective in malonate-lesioned rats, an inflammatory model of
      Huntington's disease: role of CB1 and CB2 receptors. *ACS Chem
      Neurosci* 3(5):400–6.

556. Beckman Y, Secil Y, Gungor B, Yigit T (2010) Tardive Dystonia and
      the Use of Cannabis. *Turk Psikiyatr Derg* 21(1):90–91.

557. Consroe P, et al. (1991) Controlled clinical trial of cannabidiol in
      Huntington's disease. *Pharmacol Biochem Behav* 40(3):701–8.

558. Ravikoff Allegretti J, Courtwright A, Lucci M, Korzenik JR, Levine J
      (2013) Marijuana use patterns among patients with inflammatory
      bowel disease. *Inflamm Bowel Dis* 19(13):2809–14.

559. Lahat A, Lang A, Ben-Horin S (2012) Impact of cannabis treat-
      ment on the quality of life, weight and clinical disease activity in
      inflammatory bowel disease patients: a pilot prospective study.
      Digestion 85(1):1–8.

560. Kazemi H, Rahgozar M, Speckmann E-J, Gorji A (2012) Effect of
      cannabinoid receptor activation on spreading depression. *Iran J
      Basic Med Sci* 15(4):926–36.

561. Russo E (2001) Hemp for headache: An in-depth historical and
      scientific review of cannabis in migraine treatment. *J cannabis Ther*
      1(2):21–92.

562. Akerman S, Kaube H, Goadsby PJ (2004) Anandamide is
      able to inhibit trigeminal neurons using an in vivo model of

trigeminovascular-mediated nociception. *J Pharmacol Exp Ther* 309(1):56–63.

563. el-Mallakh RS, Kranzler HR, Kamanitz JR (1991) Headaches and psychoactive substance use. *Headache* 31(9):584–7.

564. Volfe Z, Dvilansky A, Nathan I (1985) Cannabinoids block release of serotonin from platelets induced by plasma from migraine patients. *Int J Clin Pharmacol Res* 5(4):243–6.

565. Raby W, Modica P, Wolintz R, Murtaugh K (2006) Dronabinol reduces signs and symptoms of idiopathic intracranial hypertension: a case report. *J Ocul Pharmacol Ther* 22(1):68–75.

566. Robbins M, Tarshish S, Solomon S, Grosberg B (2009) Cluster Attacks Responsive to Recreational Cannabis and Dronabinol. *Headache* 49(6):914–916.

567. Evans RW, Ramadan NM Are cannabis-based chemicals helpful in headache? *Headache* 44(7):726–7.

568. Zajicek JP, et al. (2005) Cannabinoids in multiple sclerosis (CAMS) study: safety and efficacy data for 12 months follow up. *J Neurol Neurosurg Psychiatry* 76(12):1664–9.

569. Zajicek JP, Hobart JC, Slade A, Barnes D, Mattison PG (2012) Multiple sclerosis and extract of cannabis: results of the MUSEC trial. *J Neurol Neurosurg Psychiatry* 83(11):1125–32.

570. Zajicek J, et al. (2003) Cannabinoids for treatment of spasticity and other symptoms related to multiple sclerosis (CAMS study): multicentre randomised placebo-controlled trial. *Lancet* 362(9395):1517–26.

571. Fernández O (2014) Advances in the management of multiple sclerosis spasticity: recent clinical trials. *Eur Neurol* 72 Suppl 1:9–11.

572. Brunt TM, van Genugten M, Höner-Snoeken K, van de Velde MJ, Niesink RJM (2014) Therapeutic satisfaction and subjective effects of different strains of pharmaceutical-grade cannabis. *J Clin Psychopharmacol* 34(3):344–9.

573. Lu L, et al. (2012) Cost effectiveness of oromucosal cannabis-based medicine (Sativex®) for spasticity in multiple sclerosis. *Pharmacoeconomics* 30(12):1157–71.

574. Sánchez Robles EM, Bagües Arias A, Martín Fontelles MI (2012) Cannabinoids and muscular pain. Effectiveness of the local administration in rat. *Eur J Pain* 16(8):1116–27.

575. Capasso R, et al. (2011) Inhibitory effect of standardized cannabis sativa extract and its ingredient cannabidiol on rat and human bladder contractility. *Urology* 77(4):1006.e9–1006.e15.

576. Buccellato E, et al. (2011) Acute and chronic cannabinoid extracts administration affects motor function in a CREAE model of multiple sclerosis. *J Ethnopharmacol* 133(3):1033–8.

577. Koch G, et al. (2009) Cannabis-based treatment induces polarity-reversing plasticity assessed by theta burst stimulation in humans. *Brain Stimul* 2(4):229–33.

578. Thaera GM, Wellik KE, Carter JL, Demaerschalk BM, Wingerchuk DM (2009) Do cannabinoids reduce multiple sclerosis-related spasticity? *Neurologist* 15(6):369–71.

579. Martínez-Rodríguez JE, et al. (2008) Cannabis use in Spanish patients with multiple sclerosis: fulfilment of patients' expectations? *J Neurol Sci* 273(1-2):103–7.

580. Chong MS, et al. (2006) Cannabis use in patients with multiple sclerosis. *Mult Scler* 12(5):646–51.

581. Freeman RM, et al. (2006) The effect of cannabis on urge incontinence in patients with multiple sclerosis: a multicentre, randomised placebo-controlled trial (CAMS-LUTS). *Int Urogynecol J Pelvic Floor Dysfunct* 17(6):636–41.

582. Clark AJ, Ware MA, Yazer E, Murray TJ, Lynch ME (2004) Patterns of cannabis use among patients with multiple sclerosis. *Neurology* 62(11):2098–100.

583. Simmons RD, Ponsonby A-L, van der Mei IAF, Sheridan P (2004) What affects your MS? Responses to an anonymous, Internet-based epidemiological survey. *Mult Scler* 10(2):202–11.

584. Fox P, Bain PG, Glickman S, Carroll C, Zajicek J (2004) The effect of cannabis on tremor in patients with multiple sclerosis. *Neurology* 62(7):1105–9.

585. Page SA, Verhoef MJ, Stebbins RA, Metz LM, Levy JC (2003) Cannabis use as described by people with multiple sclerosis. *Can J Neurol Sci* 30(3):201–5.

586. Killestein J, et al. (2003) Immunomodulatory effects of orally administered cannabinoids in multiple sclerosis. *J Neuroimmunol* 137(1-2):140–3.

587. Dell'Osso LF (2000) Suppression of pendular nystagmus by smoking cannabis in a patient with multiple sclerosis. *Neurology* 54(11):2190–1.

588. Baker D, et al. (2000) Cannabinoids control spasticity and tremor in a multiple sclerosis model. *Nature* 404(6773):84–7.

589. Schon F, et al. (1999) Suppression of pendular nystagmus by smoking cannabis in a patient with multiple sclerosis. *Neurology* 53(9):2209–10.

590. Witting A, et al. (2006) Experimental autoimmune encephalomyelitis disrupts endocannabinoid-mediated neuroprotection. *Proc Natl Acad Sci U S A* 103(16):6362–7.

591. Hodges C (2002) Personal account of medical use of cannabis. *J Cannabis Ther* 2(3-4):155–160.

592. Kavia R, De Ridder D, Constantinescu C, Stott C, Fowler C (2010) Randomized controlled trial of Sativex to treat detrusor overactivity in multiple sclerosis. *Mult Scler* 16(11):1349–1359.

593. Page SA, Verhoef MJ (2006) Medicinal marijuana use: experiences of people with multiple sclerosis. *Can Fam Physician* 52:64–5.

594. Vicente-Valor MI, et al. (2013) Cannabis derivatives therapy for a seronegative stiff-person syndrome: a case report. *J Clin Pharm Ther* 38(1):71–3.

595. Warms CA, Turner JA, Marshall HM, Cardenas DD (2002) Treatments for chronic pain associated with spinal cord injuries: many are tried, few are helpful. *Clin J Pain* 18(3):154–63.

596. Slatkin N (2007) Cannabinoids in the treatment of chemother-apy-induced nausea and vomiting: Beyond prevention of acute emesis. *J Support Oncol* 5:1–9.

597. Roberson EK, Patrick WK, Hurwitz EL (2014) Marijuana use and maternal experiences of severe nausea during pregnancy in Hawai'i. *Hawaii J Med Public Health* 73(9):283–7.

598. Westfall RE, Janssen PA, Lucas P, Capler R (2006) Survey of medici-nal cannabis use among childbearing women: patterns of its use in pregnancy and retroactive self-assessment of its efficacy against "morning sickness". *Complement Ther Clin Pract* 12(1):27–33.

599. Mims RB, Lee JH (1977) Adverse effects of intravenous cannabis tea. *J Natl Med Assoc* 69(7):491–5.

600. Duran M, et al. (2010) Preliminary efficacy and safety of an oromu-cosal standardized cannabis extract in chemotherapy-induced nausea and vomiting. *Br J Clin Pharmacol* 70(5):656–663.

601. Ware M, Doyle C, Woods R, Lynch M, Clark A (2003) Cannabis use for chronic non-cancer pain: results of a prospective survey. *Pain* 102(1-2):211–216.

602. Ware M, Ducruet T, Robinson A (2006) Evaluation of herbal can-nabis characteristics by medical users: a randomized trial. *Harm Reduct J* 3:32.

603. Pearce DD, Mitsouras K, Irizarry KJ (2014) Discriminating the effects of Cannabis sativa and Cannabis indica: a web survey of medical cannabis users. *J Altern Complement Med* 20(10):787–91.

604. Eisenberg E, Ogintz M, Almog S (2014) The pharmacokinetics, effi-cacy, safety, and ease of use of a novel portable metered-dose cannabis inhaler in patients with chronic neuropathic pain: a phase 1a study. *J Pain Palliat Care Pharmacother* 28(3):216–25.

605. Cameron C, Watson D, Robinson J (2014) Use of a synthetic can-nabinoid in a correctional population for posttraumatic stress disorder-related insomnia and nightmares, chronic pain, harm

reduction, and other indications: a retrospective evaluation. *J Clin Psychopharmacol* 34(5):559–64.

606. Webb CW, Webb SM (2014) Therapeutic benefits of cannabis: a patient survey. *Hawaii J Med Public Health* 73(4):109–11.

607. Paula-Freire LIG, Andersen ML, Gama VS, Molska GR, Carlini ELA (2014) The oral administration of trans-caryophyllene attenuates acute and chronic pain in mice. *Phytomedicine* 21(3):356–62.

608. Schröder S, et al. (2013) Can medical herbs stimulate regeneration or neuroprotection and treat neuropathic pain in chemotherapy-induced peripheral neuropathy? *Evid Based Complement Alternat Med* 2013:423713.

609. Katsuyama S, et al. (2013) Involvement of peripheral cannabinoid and opioid receptors in β-caryophyllene-induced antinociception. *Eur J Pain* 17(5):664–75.

610. Collen M (2012) Prescribing cannabis for harm reduction. *Harm Reduct J* 9:1.

611. Aggarwal SK, et al. (2013) Prospectively surveying health-related quality of life and symptom relief in a lot-based sample of medical cannabis-using patients in urban Washington State reveals managed chronic illness and debility. *Am J Hosp Palliat Care* 30(6):523–31.

612. Bonfá L, Vinagre RC de O, de Figueiredo NV (2008) Cannabinoids in chronic pain and palliative care. *Rev Bras Anestesiol* 58(3):267–79.

613. Nguyen PT, et al. (2012) β-arrestin2 regulates cannabinoid CB1 receptor signaling and adaptation in a central nervous system region-dependent manner. *Biol Psychiatry* 71(8):714–24.

614. Ahrens J, et al. (2009) Positive allosteric modulatory effects of ajulemic acid at strychnine-sensitive glycine alpha1- and alpha1beta-receptors. *Naunyn Schmiedebergs Arch Pharmacol* 379(4):371–8.

615. Howard J, Anie K, Holdcroft A, Korn S, Davies S (2005) Cannabis use in sickle cell disease: a questionnaire study. *Br J Haematol* 131(1):123–128.

616. Russo E, et al. (2002) Chronic cannabis use in the Compassionate Investigational New Drug Program: An examination of benefits and adverse effects of legal clinical cannabis. *J cannabis Ther* 2(1):3–57.

617. Bottorff JL, Johnson JL, Moffat BM, Mulvogue T (2009) Relief-oriented use of marijuana by teens. *Subst Abuse Treat Prev Policy* 4:7.

618. Tripp DA, et al. (2014) A survey of cannabis (marijuana) use and self-reported benefit in men with chronic prostatitis/chronic pelvic pain syndrome. *Can Urol Assoc J* 8(11-12):E901–5.

619. Wallace M, et al. (2007) Dose-dependent effects of smoked cannabis on capsaicin-induced pain and hyperalgesia in healthy volunteers. *Anesthesiology* 107(5):785–796.

620. Stein MD, et al. (2015) Chronic Pain and DepressionAmong Primary Care Patients Treated with Buprenorphine. *J Gen Intern Med*.

621. Kwilasz AJ, Negus SS (2012) Dissociable effects of the cannabinoid receptor agonists Δ9-tetrahydrocannabinol and CP55940 on pain-stimulated versus pain-depressed behavior in rats. *J Pharmacol Exp Ther* 343(2):389–400.

622. Whitfield R, Bechtel L, Starich G (1997) The impact of ethanol and Marinol/marijuana usage on HIV+/AIDS patients undergoing azidothymidine, azidothymidine/dideoxycytidine, or dideoxyinosine therapy. *Alcohol Clin Exp Res* 21(1):122–127.

623. Venderová K, Růzicka E, Vorísek V, Visnovský P (2004) Survey on cannabis use in Parkinson's disease: subjective improvement of motor symptoms. *Mov Disord* 19(9):1102–6.

624. Carroll CB, et al. (2004) Cannabis for dyskinesia in Parkinson disease: a randomized double-blind crossover study. *Neurology* 63(7):1245–50.

625. Frankel J, Hughes A, Lees A, Stern G (1990) Marijuana for Parkinsonian tremor. *J Neurol Neurosurg Psychiatry* 53:436.

626. Grant I (2013) Medicinal cannabis and painful sensory neuropathy. *Virtual Mentor* 15(5):466–9.

627. Roitman P, Mechoulam R, Cooper-Kazaz R, Shalev A (2014) Preliminary, open-label, pilot study of add-on oral Δ9-tetrahydrocannabinol in chronic post-traumatic stress disorder. *Clin Drug Investig* 34(8):587–91.

628. Greer GR, Grob CS, Halberstadt AL (2014) PTSD symptom reports of patients evaluated for the New Mexico Medical Cannabis Program. *J Psychoactive Drugs* 46(1):73–7.

629. Villagonzalo K, et al. (2011) The relationship between substance use and posttraumatic stress disorder in a methadone maintenance treatment program. *Compr Psychiatry* 52(5):562–566.

630. Bonn-Miller MO, Babson KA, Vandrey R (2014) Using cannabis to help you sleep: heightened frequency of medical cannabis use among those with PTSD. *Drug Alcohol Depend* 136:162–5.

631. Gross DW, Hamm J, Ashworth NL, Quigley D (2004) Marijuana use and epilepsy: prevalence in patients of a tertiary care epilepsy center. *Neurology* 62(11):2095–7.

632. Wallace MJ, Blair RE, Falenski KW, Martin BR, DeLorenzo RJ (2003) The endogenous cannabinoid system regulates seizure frequency and duration in a model of temporal lobe epilepsy. *J Pharmacol Exp Ther* 307(1):129–37.

633. Ng SK, Brust JC, Hauser WA, Susser M (1990) Illicit drug use and the risk of new-onset seizures. *Am J Epidemiol* 132(1):47–57.

634. Johnson DD, McNeill JR, Crawford RD, Wilcox WC (1975) Epileptiform seizures in domestic fowl. V. The anticonvulsant activity of delta9-tetrahydrocannabinol. *Can J Physiol Pharmacol* 53(6):1007–13.

635. Kwiatkoski M, Guimarães FS, Del-Bel E (2012) Cannabidiol-treated rats exhibited higher motor score after cryogenic spinal cord injury. *Neurotox Res* 21(3):271–80.

636. Pugh G, Abood ME, Welch SP (1995) Antisense oligodeoxynucle-otides to the kappa-1 receptor block the antinociceptive effects of delta 9-THC in the spinal cord. *Brain Res* 689(1):157–8.

637. Dunn M, Davis R (1974) The perceived effects of marijuana on spinal cord injured males. *Paraplegia* 12:175.

638. Schweizer A, Bircher H (2009) Reposition of a dislocated shoulder under use of cannabis. *Wilderness Environ Med* 20(3):301–302.

639. Psychoyos D, Hungund B, Cooper T, Finnell RH (2008) A canna-binoid analogue of Delta9-tetrahydrocannabinol disrupts neu-ral development in chick. *Birth Defects Res B Dev Reprod Toxicol* 83(5):477–88.

640. Ceci C, Proietti Onori M, Macrì S, Laviola G (2014) Interaction Between the Endocannabinoid and Serotonergic System in the Exhibition of Head Twitch Response in Four Mouse Strains. *Neurotox Res*.

641. Müller-Vahl KR, Kolbe H, Schneider U, Emrich HM (1998) Cannabinoids: possible role in patho-physiology and therapy of Gilles de la Tourette syndrome. *Acta Psychiatr Scand* 98(6):502–6.

642. Müller-Vahl KR, et al. (2001) Influence of treatment of Tourette syndrome with delta9-tetrahydrocannabinol (delta9-THC) on neu-ropsychological performance. *Pharmacopsychiatry* 34(1):19–24.

643. Müller-Vahl KR, et al. (2002) Treatment of Tourette's syndrome with Delta 9-tetrahydrocannabinol (THC): a randomized crossover trial. *Pharmacopsychiatry* 35(2):57–61.

644. Müller-Vahl KR, et al. (2003) Delta 9-tetrahydrocannabinol (THC) is effective in the treatment of tics in Tourette syndrome: a 6-week randomized trial. *J Clin Psychiatry* 64(4):459–65.

645. Müller-Vahl KR, et al. (2003) Treatment of Tourette syndrome with delta-9-tetrahydrocannabinol (delta 9-THC): no influence on neuropsychological performance. *Neuropsychopharmacology* 28(2):384–8.

646. Hemming M, Yellowlees PM (1993) Effective treatment of Tourette's syndrome with marijuana. *J Psychopharmacol* 7(4):389–91.

647.   Sandyk R, Awerbuch G (1988) Marijuana and Tourette's Syndrome. *J Clin Psychopharmacol* 8:444–445.

648.   Elliott MB, Tuma RF, Amenta PS, Barbe MF, Jallo JI (2011) Acute effects of a selective cannabinoid-2 receptor agonist on neuroinflammation in a model of traumatic brain injury. *J Neurotrauma* 28(6):973–81.

649.   Dawson KS, Batchelor J, Meares S, Chapman J, Marosszeky JE (2007) Applicability of neural reserve theory in mild traumatic brain injury. *Brain Inj* 21(9):943–9.

650.   Ungerleider J, et al. (1985) THC or compazine for the cancer chemotherapy patient- the UCLA study. Part II: patient drug preference. *Am J Clin Oncol* 8:142–147.

651.   Artim R, DiBella N (1983) Tetrahydrocannabinol (THC) plus prochlorperazine (PCZ) for refractory nausea and vomiting (N/V). *Proc Am Soc Clin Oncol* 2:84.

652.   Gralla R, et al. (1984) Antiemetic therapy: a review of recent studies and a report of a random assignment trial comparing metoclopramide with delta-9-tetrahydrocannabinol. *Cancer Treat Rep* 68:163–172.

653.   Doblin RE, Kleiman MA (1991) Marijuana as antiemetic medicine: a survey of oncologists' experiences and attitudes. *J Clin Oncol* 9(7):1314–9.

654.   De Jong B, Prentiss D, McFarland W, Machekano R, Israelski D (2005) Marijuana use and its association with adherence to antiretroviral therapy among HIV-infected persons with moderate to severe nausea. *J Acquir Immune Defic Syndr* 38(1):43–46.

655.   Corless I, et al. (2009) Marijuana Effectiveness as an HIV Self-Care Strategy. *Clin Nurs Res* 18(2):172–193.

656.   Schwartz R, Voth E, Sheridan M (1997) Marijuana to prevent nausea and vomiting in cancer patients: a survey of clinical oncologists. *South Med J* 90(2):167–172.

657. Van Sickle MD, et al. (2001) Cannabinoids inhibit emesis through CB1 receptors in the brainstem of the ferret. *Gastroenterology* 121(4):767–74.

658. Curry W-N (2002) Hyperemesis gravidarum and clinical cannabis: To eat or not to eat? *J Cannabis Ther* 2(3-4):63–83.

659. Ngaotepprutaram T, Kaplan BLF, Kaminski NE (2013) Impaired NFAT and NFκB activation are involved in suppression of CD40 ligand expression by Δ(9)-tetrahydrocannabinol in human CD4(+) T cells. *Toxicol Appl Pharmacol* 273(1):209–18.

660. Muscaritoli M, Molfino A, Lucia S, Rossi Fanelli F (2014) Cachexia: A preventable comorbidity of cancer. A T.A.R.G.E.T. approach. *Crit Rev Oncol Hematol.*

661. Orellana-Serradell O, et al. (2015) Proapoptotic effect of endocannabinoids in prostate cancer cells. *Oncol Rep* 33(4):1599–608.

662. Sharkey KA, Darmani NA, Parker LA (2014) Regulation of nausea and vomiting by cannabinoids and the endocannabinoid system. *Eur J Pharmacol* 722:134–46.

663. Crawford S, Buckman R (1986) Nabilone and metoclopramide in the treatment of nausea and vomiting due to cisplatinum: a double blind study. *Med Oncol Tumor Pharmacother* 3:39–42.

664. Cunningham D, et al. (1988) A randomized trial of oral nabilone and prochlorperazine compared to intravenous metoclopramide and dexamethasone in the treatment of nausea and vomiting induced by chemotherapy regimens containing cisplatin or cisplatin analogues. *Eur J Cancer Clin Oncol* 24:685–689.

665. Ware MA, Doyle CR, Woods R, Lynch ME, Clark AJ (2003) Cannabis use for chronic non-cancer pain: results of a prospective survey. *Pain* 102(1-2):211–6.

666. Ryan LM, Warden DL (2003) Post concussion syndrome. *Int Rev Psychiatry* 15(4):310–6.

667. Wolkenstein P, et al. (2014) Smoking and Dietary Factors Associated with Moderate-to-Severe Acne in French Adolescents

and Young Adults: Results of a Survey Using a Representative Sample. *Dermatology*.

668. Sethi BB, et al. (1986) Antianxiety effect of cannabis: involvement of central benzodiazepine receptors. *Biol Psychiatry* 21(1):3–10.

669. Phan KL, et al. (2008) Cannabinoid modulation of amygdala reactivity to social signals of threat in humans. *J Neurosci* 28(10):2313–9.

670. Nardo M, Casarotto PC, Gomes F V, Guimarães FS (2014) Cannabidiol reverses the mCPP-induced increase in marble-burying behavior. *Fundam Clin Pharmacol* 28(5):544–50.

671. Degenhardt L, Hall W, Lynskey M (2001) The relationship between cannabis use, depression and anxiety among Australian adults: findings from the National Survey of Mental Health and Well-Being. *Soc Psychiatry Psychiatr Epidemiol* 36(5):219–27.

672. Dumas P, et al. (2002) Cannabis use correlates with schizotypal personality traits in healthy students. *Psychiatry Res* 109(1):27–35.

673. Zvolensky MJ, et al. (2008) Prospective associations between cannabis use, abuse, and dependence and panic attacks and disorder. *J Psychiatr Res* 42(12):1017–23.

674. Tournier M, Sorbara F, Gindre C, Swendsen JD, Verdoux H (2003) Cannabis use and anxiety in daily life: a naturalistic investigation in a non-clinical population. *Psychiatry Res* 118(1):1–8.

675. Gregg JM, Small EW, Moore R, Raft D, Toomey TC (1976) Emotional response to intravenous delta9tetrahydrocannabinol during oral surgery. *J Oral Surg* 34(4):301–13.

676. Tashkin D, Shapiro B, Frank I (1974) Acute effects of smoked marijuana and oral delta9-tetrahydrocannabinol on specific airway conductance in asthmatic subjects. *Am Rev Respir Dis* 109(4):420–428.

677. Tashkin DP, Shapiro BJ, Lee YE, Harper CE (1975) Effects of smoked marijuana in experimentally induced asthma. *Am Rev Respir Dis* 112(3):377–86.

678. Vachon L, Mikus P, Morrissey W, FitzGerald M, Gaensler E (1976) Bronchial effect of marihuana smoke in asthma. *The Pharmacology of Marihuana*, eds Braude M, Szara S (Raven Press, New York), pp 777–784.

679. Steffens S, et al. (2005) Low dose oral cannabinoid therapy reduces progression of atherosclerosis in mice. *Nature* 434(7034):782–6.

680. Takeda S, et al. (2011) Δ9-tetrahydrocannabinol and its major metabolite Δ9-tetrahydrocannabinol-11-oic acid as 15-lipoxygenase inhibitors. *J Pharm Sci* 100(3):1206–11.

681. Cornicelli JA, Gilman SR, Krom BA, Kottke BA (1981) Cannabinoids impair the formation of cholesteryl ester in cultured human cells. *Arteriosclerosis* 1(6):449–54.

682. Callaway J, et al. (2005) Efficacy of dietary hempseed oil in patients with atopic dermatitis. *J Dermatolog Treat* 16(2):87–94.

683. Aharonovich E, et al. (2006) Concurrent cannabis use during treatment for comorbid ADHD and cocaine dependence: effects on outcome. *Am J Drug Alcohol Abuse* 32(4):629–635.

684. O'Connell T, Bou-Matar C (2007) Long term marijuana users seeking medical cannabis in California (2001-2007): demographics, social characteristics, patterns of cannabis and other drug use of 4117 applicants. *Harm Reduct J* 4:16.

685. Silva N, et al. (2014) Searching for a neurobiological basis for self-medication theory in ADHD comorbid with substance use disorders: an in vivo study of dopamine transporters using (99m) Tc-TRODAT-1 SPECT. *Clin Nucl Med* 39(2):e129–34.

686. Grinspoon L, Bakalar J (1998) The use of cannabis as a mood stabilizer in bipolar disorder: anecdotal evidence and the need for clinical research. *J Psychoactive Drugs* 30(2):171–177.

687. Ringen PA, et al. (2010) Opposite relationships between cannabis use and neurocognitive functioning in bipolar disorder and schizophrenia. *Psychol Med* 40(8):1337–47.

688. Braga RJ, Burdick KE, Derosse P, Malhotra AK (2012) Cognitive and clinical outcomes associated with cannabis use in patients with bipolar I disorder. *Psychiatry Res* 200(2-3):242–5.

689. Valvassori SS, et al. (2011) Effects of cannabidiol on amphetamine-induced oxidative stress generation in an animal model of mania. *J Psychopharmacol* 25(2):274–80.

690. Feingold D, Weiser M, Rehm J, Lev-Ran S (2014) The association between cannabis use and mood disorders: A longitudinal study. *J Affect Disord* 172C:211–218.

691. Ranney DN, et al. (2009) Marijuana use in potential liver transplant candidates. *Am J Transplant* 9(2):280–5.

692. Pickering EE, et al. (2011) Cannabinoid effects on ventilation and breathlessness: a pilot study of efficacy and safety. *Chron Respir Dis* 8(2):109–18.

693. Tan WC, et al. (2009) Marijuana and chronic obstructive lung disease: a population-based study. *CMAJ* 180(8):814–20.

694. Fiorelli A, et al. (2014) Does cannabis smoking predispose to lung bulla formation? *Asian Cardiovasc Thorac Ann* 22(1):65–71.

695. Tashkin DP, Simmons MS, Sherrill DL, Coulson AH (1997) Heavy habitual marijuana smoking does not cause an accelerated decline in FEV1 with age. *Am J Respir Crit Care Med* 155(1):141–8.

696. Dreher M (20025) Crack heads and roots daughters: The therapeutic use of cannabis in Jamaica. *J cannabis Ther* 2(3-4):121–133.

697. González-Cuevas G, et al. (2007) Subchronic cannabinoid agonist (WIN 55,212-2) treatment during cocaine abstinence alters subsequent cocaine seeking behavior. *Neuropsychopharmacology* 32(11):2260–6.

698. Silveira JW, et al. (2014) Protective effects of cannabidiol on lesion-induced intervertebral disc degeneration. *PLoS One* 9(12):e113161.

699. Farris SG, Zvolensky MJ, Boden MT, Bonn-Miller MO (2014) Cannabis use expectancies mediate the relation between depressive symptoms and cannabis use among cannabis-dependent veterans. *J Addict Med* 8(2):130–6.

700. Ware M, Adams H, Guy G (2005) The medicinal use of cannabis in the UK: results of a nationwide survey. *Int J Clin Pharmacol Res* 59(3):291–295.

701. Aselton P (2012) Sources of stress and coping in American college students who have been diagnosed with depression. *J Child Adolesc Psychiatr Nurs* 25(3):119–23.

702. Manrique-Garcia E, Zammit S, Dalman C, Hemmingsson T, Allebeck P (2012) Cannabis use and depression: a longitudinal study of a national cohort of Swedish conscripts. *BMC Psychiatry* 12:112.

703. Chabrol H, Melioli T, Goutaudier N (2014) Cannabis use and suicidal ideations in high-school students. *Addict Behav* 39(12):1766–8.

704. Hooshmand S, Willoughby T, Good M (2012) Does the direction of effects in the association between depressive symptoms and health-risk behaviors differ by behavior? A longitudinal study across the high school years. *J Adolesc Health* 50(2):140–7.

705. Griffith-Lendering MFH, Huijbregts SCJ, Mooijaart A, Vollebergh WAM, Swaab H (2011) Cannabis use and development of externalizing and internalizing behaviour problems in early adolescence: A TRAILS study. *Drug Alcohol Depend* 116(1-3):11–7.

706. De Graaf R, et al. (2010) Early cannabis use and estimated risk of later onset of depression spells: Epidemiologic evidence from the population-based World Health Organization World Mental Health Survey Initiative. *Am J Epidemiol* 172(2):149–59.

707. Mariani JJ, Haney M, Hart CL, Vosburg SK, Levin FR (2009) Effects of research setting on observed depressive symptoms in marijuana users. *J Subst Abuse Treat* 37(4):431–4.

708. Pedersen W (2008) Does cannabis use lead to depression and suicidal behaviours? A population-based longitudinal study. *Acta Psychiatr Scand* 118(5):395–403.

709. Harder VS, Stuart EA, Anthony JC (2008) Adolescent cannabis problems and young adult depression: male-female stratified propensity score analyses. *Am J Epidemiol* 168(6):592–601.

710. Leventhal AM, Lewinsohn PM, Pettit JW (2008) Prospective relations between melancholia and substance use disorders. *Am J Drug Alcohol Abuse* 34(3):259–67.

711. Harder VS, Morral AR, Arkes J (2006) Marijuana use and depression among adults: Testing for causal associations. *Addiction* 101(10):1463–72.

712. Green BE, Ritter C (2000) Marijuana use and depression. *J Health Soc Behav* 41(1):40–9.

713. Rajavashisth TB, et al. (2012) Decreased prevalence of diabetes in marijuana users: cross-sectional data from the National Health and Nutrition Examination Survey (NHANES) III. *BMJ Open* 2:e000494.

714. Gallant M, Odei-Addo F, Frost CL, Levendal R-A (2009) Biological effects of THC and a lipophilic cannabis extract on normal and insulin resistant 3T3-L1 adipocytes. *Phytomedicine* 16(10):942–9.

715. Nalin DR, et al. (1978) Cannabis, hypochlorhydria, and cholera. *Lancet* 2(8095):859–62.

716. Huy ND, Belleau R, Roy PE (1975) Toxicity of marijuana and tobacco smoking in the beagle. *Int J Clin Pharmacol Biopharm* 12(1-2):267–76.

717. Gilson I, Busalacchi M (1998) Marijuana for intractable hiccup. *Lancet* 351(9098):267.

718. Vandrey R, Umbricht A, Strain E (2011) Increased Blood Pressure Following Abrupt Cessation of Daily Cannabis Use. *J Addict Med* 5(1):16–20.

719. Misra DP, Kiely JL (1995) The effect of smoking on the risk of gestational hypertension. *Early Hum Dev* 40(2):95–107.

720. Dwivedi S, Kumar V, Aggarwal A (2008) Cannabis smoking and acute coronary syndrome: two illustrative cases. *Int J Cardiol* 128(2):e54–7.

721. Merzouki A, Mesa JM (2002) Concerning kif, a Cannabis sativa L. preparation smoked in the Rif mountains of northern Morocco. *J Ethnopharmacol* 81(3):403–6.

722. Pradeep A, Thomas S, Roberts EO, Proudlock FA, Gottlob I Reduction of congenital nystagmus in a patient after smoking cannabis. *Strabismus* 16(1):29–32.

723. Brook JS, Lee JY, Finch SJ, Balka EB, Brook DW (2013) Physical factors, personal characteristics, and substance use: associations with obesity. *Subst Abus* 34(3):273–6.

724. Riedel G, et al. (2009) Synthetic and plant-derived cannabinoid receptor antagonists show hypophagic properties in fasted and non-fasted mice. *Br J Pharmacol* 156(7):1154–66.

725. Hine B, Torrelio M, Gershon S (1975) Differential effect of cannabinol and cannabidiol on THC-induced responses during abstinence in morphine-dependent rats. *Res Commun Chem Pathol Pharmacol* 12(1):185–8.

726. Nava F, Manzato E, Lucchini A (2007) Chronic cannabis use does not affect the normalization of hypothalamic-pituitary-adrenal (HPA) axis induced by methadone in heroin addicts. *Prog Neuropsychopharmacol Biol Psychiatry* 31(5):1089–94.

727. Solinas M, Panlilio L V, Goldberg SR (2004) Exposure to delta-9-tetrahydrocannabinol (THC) increases subsequent heroin taking but not heroin's reinforcing efficacy: a self-administration study in rats. *Neuropsychopharmacology* 29(7):1301–11.

728. Weizman T, Gelkopf M, Melamed Y, Adelson M, Bleich A Cannabis abuse is not a risk factor for treatment outcome in methadone maintenance treatment: a 1-year prospective study in an Israeli clinic. *Aust N Z J Psychiatry* 38(1-2):42–6.

729. Epstein DH, Preston KL (2003) Does cannabis use predict poor outcome for heroin-dependent patients on maintenance treatment? Past findings and more evidence against. *Addiction* 98(3):269–79.

730. Budney AJ, Bickel WK, Amass L (1998) Marijuana use and treatment outcome among opioid-dependent patients. *Addiction* 93(4):493–503.

731. Kraft B, et al. (2008) Lack of analgesia by oral standardized cannabis extract on acute inflammatory pain and hyperalgesia in volunteers. *Anesthesiology* 109(1):101–110.

732. Hill S, Schwin R, Goodwin D, Powell B (1974) Marihuana and pain. *J Pharmacol Exp Ther* 188:415–418.

733. Wilkinson JD, Williamson EM (2007) Cannabinoids inhibit human keratinocyte proliferation through a non-CB1/CB2 mechanism and have a potential therapeutic value in the treatment of psoriasis. *J Dermatol Sci* 45(2):87–92.

734. Arseneault L, Cannon M, Witton J, Murray RM (2004) Causal association between cannabis and psychosis: examination of the evidence. *Br J Psychiatry* 184:110–7.

735. Schubart CD, et al. (2011) Cannabis with high cannabidiol content is associated with fewer psychotic experiences. *Schizophr Res* 130(1-3):216–21.

736. Burns JK, Jhazbhay K, Emsley R (2010) Cannabis use predicts shorter duration of untreated psychosis and lower levels of negative symptoms in first-episode psychosis: a South African study. *Afr J Psychiatry* 13(5):395–9.

737. Coulston CM, Perdices M, Tennant CC (2007) The neuropsychological correlates of cannabis use in schizophrenia: lifetime abuse/dependence, frequency of use, and recency of use. *Schizophr Res* 96(1-3):169–84.

738. Dixon L, Haas G, Weiden PJ, Sweeney J, Frances AJ (1991) Drug abuse in schizophrenic patients: clinical correlates and reasons for use. *Am J Psychiatry* 148(2):224–30.

739. Mueser KT, et al. (1990) Prevalence of substance abuse in schizophrenia: demographic and clinical correlates. *Schizophr Bull* 16(1):31–56.

740. Koola MM, et al. (2012) Alcohol and cannabis use and mortality in people with schizophrenia and related psychotic disorders. *J Psychiatr Res* 46(8):987–93.

741. Schnell T, Kleiman A, Gouzoulis-Mayfrank E, Daumann J, Becker B (2012) Increased gray matter density in patients with schizophrenia and cannabis use: a voxel-based morphometric study using DARTEL. *Schizophr Res* 138(2-3):183–7.

742. Rabin RA, Zakzanis KK, George TP (2011) The effects of cannabis use on neurocognition in schizophrenia: a meta-analysis. *Schizophr Res* 128(1-3):111–6.

743. Rodríguez-Sánchez JM, et al. (2010) Cannabis use and cognitive functioning in first-episode schizophrenia patients. *Schizophr Res* 124(1-3):142–51.

744. Yücel M, et al. (2012) The impact of cannabis use on cognitive functioning in patients with schizophrenia: a meta-analysis of existing findings and new data in a first-episode sample. *Schizophr Bull* 38(2):316–30.

745. DeRosse P, Kaplan A, Burdick KE, Lencz T, Malhotra AK (2010) Cannabis use disorders in schizophrenia: effects on cognition and symptoms. *Schizophr Res* 120(1-3):95–100.

746. Løberg E-M, Hugdahl K (2009) Cannabis use and cognition in schizophrenia. *Front Hum Neurosci* 3:53.

747. Long LE, Malone DT, Taylor DA (2006) Cannabidiol reverses MK-801-induced disruption of prepulse inhibition in mice. *Neuropsychopharmacology* 31(4):795–803.

748. Niehaus DJH, et al. (2008) Predictors of abnormal involuntary movement in an african schizophrenia population. *J Neuropsychiatry Clin Neurosci* 20(3):317–26.

749. Ruiz-Veguilla M, et al. (2009) Fewer neurological soft signs among first episode psychosis patients with heavy cannabis use. *Schizophr Res* 107(2-3):158–64.

750. Costain WF (2008) The effects of cannabis abuse on the symptoms of schizophrenia: patient perspectives. *Int J Ment Health Nurs* 17(4):227–35.

751. Potvin S, Joyal CC, Pelletier J, Stip E (2008) Contradictory cognitive capacities among substance-abusing patients with schizophrenia: a meta-analysis. *Schizophr Res* 100(1-3):242–51.

752. Potvin S, Sepehry AA, Stip E (2006) A meta-analysis of negative symptoms in dual diagnosis schizophrenia. *Psychol Med* 36(4):431–40.

753. Jockers-Scherübl MC, et al. (2007) Cannabis induces different cognitive changes in schizophrenic patients and in healthy controls. *Prog Neuropsychopharmacol Biol Psychiatry* 31(5):1054–63.

754. Compton MT, Furman AC, Kaslow NJ (2004) Lower negative symptom scores among cannabis-dependent patients with schizophrenia-spectrum disorders: preliminary evidence from an African American first-episode sample. *Schizophr Res* 71(1):61–4.

755. Peralta V, Cuesta MJ (1992) Influence of cannabis abuse on schizophrenic psychopathology. *Acta Psychiatr Scand* 85(2):127–30.

756. Krysta K, et al. (2012) Inferior performance on selected neuropsychological tests in abstinent schizophrenia patients who have used cannabis. *Med Sci Monit* 18(9):CR581–6.

757. Herzig DA, et al. (2014) Hemispheric Language Asymmetry in First Episode Psychosis and Schizotypy: The Role of Cannabis Consumption and Cognitive Disorganization. *Schizophr Bull.*

758. Wobrock T, et al. (2007) Comorbid substance abuse and neurocognitive function in recent-onset schizophrenia. *Eur Arch Psychiatry Clin Neurosci* 257(4):203–10.

759. Dragogna F, et al. (2014) Brain Metabolism in Substance-Induced Psychosis and Schizophrenia: A Preliminary PET Study. *Neuropsychobiology* 70(4):195–202.

760. McLoughlin BC, et al. (2014) Cannabis and schizophrenia. *Cochrane database Syst Rev* 10:CD004837.

761. Power RA, et al. (2014) Genetic predisposition to schizophrenia associated with increased use of cannabis. *Mol Psychiatry* 19(11):1201–4.

762. Proal AC, Fleming J, Galvez-Buccollini JA, Delisi LE (2014) A controlled family study of cannabis users with and without psychosis. *Schizophr Res* 152(1):283–8.

763. Bugra H, et al. (2013) Cannabis use and cognitive functions in at-risk mental state and first episode psychosis. *Psychopharmacology (Berl)* 230(2):299–308.

764. Shrivastava A, Johnston M, Terpstra K, Bureau Y (2013) Pathways to Psychosis in Cannabis Abuse. *Clin Schizophr Relat Psychoses*:1–18.

765. Faber G, et al. (2012) Continued cannabis use and outcome in first-episode psychosis: data from a randomized, open-label, controlled trial. *J Clin Psychiatry* 73(5):632–8.

766. Van Dijk D, Koeter MWJ, Hijman R, Kahn RS, van den Brink W (2012) Effect of cannabis use on the course of schizophrenia in male patients: a prospective cohort study. *Schizophr Res* 137(1-3):50–7.

767. Cohen M, et al. (2012) Cerebellar grey-matter deficits, cannabis use and first-episode schizophrenia in adolescents and young adults. *Int J Neuropsychopharmacol* 15(3):297–307.

768. Sevy S, et al. (2010) Are cannabis use disorders associated with an earlier age at onset of psychosis? A study in first episode schizophrenia. *Schizophr Res* 120(1-3):101–7.

769. Scholes KE, Martin-Iverson MT (2010) Cannabis use and neuropsychological performance in healthy individuals and patients with schizophrenia. *Psychol Med* 40(10):1635–46.

770. Dekker N, et al. (2010) Cannabis use and callosal white matter structure and integrity in recent-onset schizophrenia. *Psychiatry Res* 181(1):51–6.

771. Wobrock T, Sittinger H, Behrendt B, D'Amelio R, Falkai P (2009) Comorbid substance abuse and brain morphology in recent-onset psychosis. *Eur Arch Psychiatry Clin Neurosci* 259(1):28–36.

772. Boydell J, et al. (2007) A comparison of symptoms and family history in schizophrenia with and without prior cannabis use:

implications for the concept of cannabis psychosis. *Schizophr Res* 93(1-3):203–10.

773. Dubertret C, Bidard I, Adès J, Gorwood P (2006) Lifetime positive symptoms in patients with schizophrenia and cannabis abuse are partially explained by co-morbid addiction. *Schizophr Res* 86(1-3):284–90.

774. Goswami S, Singh G, Mattoo SK, Basu D (2003) Courses of substance use and schizophrenia in the dual-diagnosis patients: is there a relationship? *Indian J Med Sci* 57(8):338–46.

775. Bersani G, Orlandi V, Gherardelli S, Pancheri P (2002) Cannabis and neurological soft signs in schizophrenia: absence of relationship and influence on psychopathology. *Psychopathology* 35(5):289–95.

776. Assies J, et al. (2001) Significantly reduced docosahexaenoic and docosapentaenoic acid concentrations in erythrocyte membranes from schizophrenic patients compared with a carefully matched control group. *Biol Psychiatry* 49(6):510–22.

777. Brunette MF, Mueser KT, Xie H, Drake RE (1997) Relationships between symptoms of schizophrenia and substance abuse. *J Nerv Ment Dis* 185(1):13–20.

778. Mathers DC, Ghodse AH (1992) Cannabis and psychotic illness. *Br J Psychiatry* 161:648–53.

779. Giordano GN, Ohlsson H, Sundquist K, Sundquist J, Kendler KS (2014) The association between cannabis abuse and subsequent schizophrenia: a Swedish national co-relative control study. *Psychol Med*:1–8.

780. Van der Meer FJ, Velthorst E, Meijer CJ, Machielsen MWJ, de Haan L (2012) Cannabis use in patients at clinical high risk of psychosis: impact on prodromal symptoms and transition to psychosis. *Curr Pharm Des* 18(32):5036–44.

781. Pencer A, Addington J (2003) Substance use and cognition in early psychosis. *J Psychiatry Neurosci* 28(1):48–54.

782.	Auther AM, et al. (2015) Alcohol confounds relationship between cannabis misuse and psychosis conversion in a high-risk sample. *Acta Psychiatr Scand.*

783.	Epstein KA, Kumra S (2014) Executive attention impairment in adolescents with schizophrenia who have used cannabis. *Schizophr Res* 157(1-3):48–54.

784.	Suárez-Pinilla P, López-Gil J, Crespo-Facorro B (2014) Immune system: a possible nexus between cannabinoids and psychosis. *Brain Behav Immun* 40:269–82.

785.	Zamberletti E, et al. (2014) Alterations of prefrontal cortex GABAergic transmission in the complex psychotic-like phenotype induced by adolescent delta-9-tetrahydrocannabinol exposure in rats. *Neurobiol Dis* 63:35–47.

786.	Raver SM, Haughwout SP, Keller A (2013) Adolescent cannabinoid exposure permanently suppresses cortical oscillations in adult mice. *Neuropsychopharmacology* 38(12):2338–47.

787.	Fernandez-Egea E, et al. (2013) Cannabis use is associated with increased CCL11 plasma levels in young healthy volunteers. *Prog Neuropsychopharmacol Biol Psychiatry* 46:25–8.

788.	Welch KA, et al. (2013) Tensor-based morphometry of cannabis use on brain structure in individuals at elevated genetic risk of schizophrenia. *Psychol Med* 43(10):2087–96.

789.	San L, Bernardo M, Gómez A, Peña M (2013) Factors associated with relapse in patients with schizophrenia. *Int J Psychiatry Clin Pract* 17(1):2–9.

790.	Kumra S, et al. (2012) Parietal lobe volume deficits in adolescents with schizophrenia and adolescents with cannabis use disorders. *J Am Acad Child Adolesc Psychiatry* 51(2):171–80.

791.	Ho B-C, Wassink TH, Ziebell S, Andreasen NC (2011) Cannabinoid receptor 1 gene polymorphisms and marijuana misuse interactions on white matter and cognitive deficits in schizophrenia. *Schizophr Res* 128(1-3):66–75.

792. Leeson VC, Harrison I, Ron MA, Barnes TRE, Joyce EM (2012) The effect of cannabis use and cognitive reserve on age at onset and psychosis outcomes in first-episode schizophrenia. *Schizophr Bull* 38(4):873–80.

793. Decoster J, et al. (2011) Age at onset of psychotic disorder: cannabis, BDNF Val66Met, and sex-specific models of gene-environment interaction. *Am J Med Genet B Neuropsychiatr Genet* 156B(3):363–9.

794. Estrada G, et al. (2011) Cannabis use and age at onset of psychosis: further evidence of interaction with COMT Val158Met polymorphism. *Acta Psychiatr Scand* 123(6):485–92.

795. Morrison PD, Stone JM (2011) Synthetic delta-9-tetrahydrocannabinol elicits schizophrenia-like negative symptoms which are distinct from sedation. *Hum Psychopharmacol* 26(1):77–80.

796. Rais M, et al. (2010) Cannabis use and progressive cortical thickness loss in areas rich in CB1 receptors during the first five years of schizophrenia. *Eur Neuropsychopharmacol* 20(12):855–65.

797. Morgan CJA, Rothwell E, Atkinson H, Mason O, Curran HV (2010) Hyper-priming in cannabis users: a naturalistic study of the effects of cannabis on semantic memory function. *Psychiatry Res* 176(2-3):213–8.

798. Stirling J, et al. (2008) Cannabis-induced psychotic-like experiences are predicted by high schizotypy. Confirmation of preliminary results in a large cohort. *Psychopathology* 41(6):371–8.

799. Roser P, et al. (2008) Effects of acute oral Delta9-tetrahydrocannabinol and standardized cannabis extract on the auditory P300 event-related potential in healthy volunteers. *Eur Neuropsychopharmacol* 18(8):569–77.

800. Veling W, Mackenbach JP, van Os J, Hoek HW (2008) Cannabis use and genetic predisposition for schizophrenia: a case-control study. *Psychol Med* 38(9):1251–6.

801. Jockers-Scherübl MC, et al. (2003) Chronic cannabis abuse raises nerve growth factor serum concentrations in drug-naive schizophrenic patients. *J Psychopharmacol* 17(4):439–45.

802. Voruganti LN, Slomka P, Zabel P, Mattar A, Awad AG (2001) Cannabis induced dopamine release: an in-vivo SPECT study. *Psychiatry Res* 107(3):173–7.

803. Dean B, Sundram S, Bradbury R, Scarr E, Copolov D (2001) Studies on [3H]CP-55940 binding in the human central nervous system: regional specific changes in density of cannabinoid-1 receptors associated with schizophrenia and cannabis use. *Neuroscience* 103(1):9–15.

804. Allebeck P, Adamsson C, Engström A, Rydberg U (1993) Cannabis and schizophrenia: a longitudinal study of cases treated in Stockholm County. *Acta Psychiatr Scand* 88(1):21–4.

805. Knudsen P, Vilmar T (1984) Cannabis and neuroleptic agents in schizophrenia. *Acta Psychiatr Scand* 69(2):162–74.

806. Treffert DA (1978) Marijuana use in schizophrenia: a clear hazard. *Am J Psychiatry* 135(10):1213–5.

807. Van der Meer FJ, Velthorst E (2015) Course of cannabis use and clinical outcome in patients with non-affective psychosis: a 3-year follow-up study. *Psychol Med*:1–12.

808. Ermis A, et al. The Relationship Between Catechol-O-Methyltransferase Gene Val158Met (COMT) Polymorphism and Premorbid Cannabis Use in Turkish Male Patients with Schizophrenia. *In Vivo* 29(1):129–132.

809. Knight-Madden J, Lewis N, Hambleton IR (2006) The prevalence of marijuana smoking in young adults with sickle cell disease: a longitudinal study. *West Indian Med J* 55(4):224–7.

810. Babson KA, Boden MT, Harris AH, Stickle TR, Bonn-Miller MO (2013) Poor sleep quality as a risk factor for lapse following a cannabis quit attempt. *J Subst Abuse Treat* 44(4):438–43.

811. Babson KA, Boden MT, Bonn-Miller MO (2013) The impact of perceived sleep quality and sleep efficiency/duration on cannabis use during a self-guided quit attempt. *Addict Behav* 38(11):2707–13.

812. Mijangos-Moreno S, Poot-Aké A, Arankowsky-Sandoval G, Murillo-Rodríguez E (2014) Intrahypothalamic injection of cannabidiol increases the extracellular levels of adenosine in nucleus accumbens in rats. *Neurosci Res* 84:60–3.

813. Gorelick DA, et al. (2013) Around-the-clock oral THC effects on sleep in male chronic daily cannabis smokers. *Am J Addict* 22(5):510–4.

814. Murillo-Rodríguez E, Palomero-Rivero M, Millán-Aldaco D, Mechoulam R, Drucker-Colín R (2011) Effects on sleep and dopamine levels of microdialysis perfusion of cannabidiol into the lateral hypothalamus of rats. *Life Sci* 88(11-12):504–11.

815. Murillo-Rodríguez E, Millán-Aldaco D, Palomero-Rivero M, Mechoulam R, Drucker-Colín R (2006) Cannabidiol, a constituent of Cannabis sativa, modulates sleep in rats. *FEBS Lett* 580(18):4337–45.

816. Murillo-Rodríguez E, Millán-Aldaco D, Palomero-Rivero M, Mechoulam R, Drucker-Colín R (2008) The nonpsychoactive Cannabis constituent cannabidiol is a wake-inducing agent. *Behav Neurosci* 122(6):1378–82.

817. Adams PM, Barratt ES (1975) Effect of chronic marijuana administration of stages of primate sleep-wakefulness. *Biol Psychiatry* 10(3):315–22.

818. Crippa JAS, et al. (2011) Neural basis of anxiolytic effects of cannabidiol (CBD) in generalized social anxiety disorder: a preliminary report. *J Psychopharmacol* 25(1):121–30.

819. Idro R, Marsh K, John CC, Newton CRJ (2010) Cerebral malaria: mechanisms of brain injury and strategies for improved neurocognitive outcome. *Pediatr Res* 68(4):267–74.

820. Roy PE, Magnan-Lapointe F, Huy ND, Boutet M (1976) Chronic inhalation of marijuana and tobacco in dogs: pulmonary pathology. *Res Commun Chem Pathol Pharmacol* 14(2):305–17.

821.   Arvin A, et al. (2007) Human Herpesviruses. Available at: http://www.ncbi.nlm.nih.gov/books/NBK47376/ [Accessed February 7, 2015].

822.   Albrecht H, Stellbrink H (1994) Hiccups in people with AIDS. *J Acquir Immune Defic Syndr* 7:735.

823.   Filbey FM, et al. (2014) Long-term effects of marijuana use on the brain. *Proc Natl Acad Sci* 111(47):16913–8.

824.   D'Souza DC, et al. (2005) Delta-9-tetrahydrocannabinol effects in schizophrenia: implications for cognition, psychosis, and addiction. *Biol Psychiatry* 57(6):594–608.